Health Care Managers in Transition

Wendy Leebov
Gail Scott

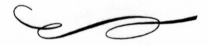

Health Care Managers in Transition

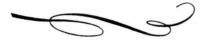

Shifting Roles and Changing Organizations

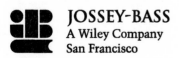

JOSSEY-BASS
A Wiley Company
San Francisco

Published by Jossey-Bass
A Wiley Imprint
989 Market Street, San Francisco, CA 94103-1741   www.josseybass.com

The Albert Einstein Healthcare Foundation has granted permission to reprint the "Service Culture Audit," © 1987; the "Model for Communicating New Expectations," © 1988; and the "Blueprint for Making Your Case," which is from Module 2 of the Service Management Essentials Program, © 1988.

Readers should be aware that Internet Web sites offered as citations and/or sources for further information may have changed or disappeared between the time this was written and when it is read.

Jossey-Bass books and products are available through most bookstores. To contact Jossey-Bass directly call our Customer Care Department within the U.S. at 800-956-7739, outside the U.S. at 317 572-3986, or fax 317-572-4002.

Jossey-Bass also publishes its books in a variety of electronic formats. Some content that appears in print may not be available in electronic books.

Library of Congress Cataloging-in-Publication Data

Leebov, Wendy.
    Health care managers in transition : shifting roles and changing organizations / Wendy Leebov, Gail Scott.
        p.   cm. — (The Jossey-Bass health series)
    Includes bibliographical references.
    ISBN 1-55542-248-9 (alk. paper)
    1. Health services administration.   I. Scott, Gail, date.
    II. Title.   III. Series
    RA971.L37   1990
    362.1'068—dc20   90-38789

Printed in the United States of America
FIRST EDITION
HB Printing   15 14 13 12 11

The Jossey-Bass Health Series

Contents

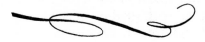

Preface

All rapids and no calm. That is the health care industry today. Competition, funding constraints, rising consumer expectations, strain between providers and payers, alternative delivery systems, and a changing work force interact to trigger dramatic changes in every health care organization's agenda and every health care employee's job. In the face of this turbulence, health care leaders have initiated far-reaching, organizationwide change efforts in order to reposition their organizations for a secure and successful future. They have launched myriad strategies to improve service, quality, productivity, management performance, employee retention, and much more.

Whatever the particular change desired, the road to change has been rocky. Many strategies have bred resistance because they have been ill conceived, insulting, or superficial. Others have fizzled due to lack of tangible senior management commitment. Still others have had minimal impact or endurance due to insufficient or ineffective follow-through. But a major cause of disappointing results has to do with managers' resistance to change.

Our group, The Einstein Consulting Group, a subsidiary of the Albert Einstein Healthcare Foundation in Philadelphia, has helped more than 170 health care organizations institute change and has witnessed a variety of sweeping change efforts in many other organizations as well. On the basis of our rich education at the "school of hard knocks," we have come to conclude that the management role and management performance are pivotal. We maintain that, regardless of how enthusiastic line employees are (and they are often very enthusiastic when faced with the need and opportunity to change), change does not take hold unless managers at every level of the organization embrace the change and help their people ride the rapids. If managers want to make things happen, they can. If they cling to obsolete practices, they can paralyze even the most ambitious effort to change.

This book is designed to make explicit and examine in depth the role shifts required of managers in the face of inevitable and unavoidable change, so that managers, for their own sakes and for the good of their organizations, will drive change, not impede it. To date, in health care, these role shifts have not been made explicit.

We interviewed hospital executives with respect to their satisfaction with managers in their organizations. Then we held a series of focus group meetings among managers in which we defined the problem as follows:

- Executives want managers throughout their organizations to change their approaches to management. They strongly feel that the management practices that once spelled success no longer work.
- Managers themselves feel the pressure to change. Once they felt successful, but now many feel inadequate, frustrated, and disillusioned because they are working so hard without appreciation.
- Neither executives nor managers are clear as to how they want managers to perform. Their new role expectations are undefined and elusive.

- Executives are frustrated because managers are not meeting new role demands, and managers are frustrated because they would try to meet the demands if only someone would tell them what they are.

On the basis of this input from executives and managers, we defined a series of role shifts that we tested with more than twelve management teams in our management team renewal retreat called "The New Vital Manager." As a result of the questions and concerns voiced, we refined our material into a list of ten role shifts that are agreeable to both managers and executives.

These ten role shifts and the practical strategies managers can use to make these shifts form the crux of this book. Once these shifts are made clear, health care managers and executives can better mobilize and support one another in adopting a management style that serves the organization and enables employees to contribute actively to organizational success.

The Book's Uniqueness

This book makes a unique contribution to the field. First of all, it focuses on health care management, not management in general. Until now, no other book has provided a down-to-earth framework for how the health care manager's role must change. While other books discuss the evolving management role, they do not acknowledge the uniqueness of health care and the revolution needed in our industry in particular.

Second, this book goes beyond rhetoric to describe how the pivotal role shifts look in realistic case situations like the ones managers face daily.

Third, the strategies for helping fulfill demanding new role expectations are fresh and new. Beyond simply labeling the shifts, we provide personal change strategies to use at will to execute shifts in attitudes and behavior. These how-to strategies are described in user-friendly detail.

Audience

We have written this book for managers at all levels in health care organizations: department heads, physician chiefs, nurse managers, product line managers, assistant vice-presidents, and vice-presidents. It will help them assess their styles and identify the role changes they need to make to cultivate the hardiness, commitment, and effectiveness that enhance both their value to their organizations and their own job satisfaction.

We have also targeted health care executives who want to build a powerhouse management team. The book will help leaders clarify and articulate their expectations to managers and identify and provide the kinds of support necessary for making the difficult transition.

For consultants, training professionals, organizational change specialists, and professors of health care management, this book serves as an ideal framework for management development and provides substantive strategies that translate rhetoric into practice. We know from experience that an entire management development curriculum can be built on this book. Finally, people considering health care management as a profession can use this book to obtain a realistic job preview—to catch a glimpse of what the job of the health care manager will entail for many years to come.

Overview of the Contents

Specifically, in each chapter, we provide a brief survey to use for self-assessment, we define the role shift in terms of the mindset and behavior involved, and we distinguish between "old" and "new" behavior in realistic case situations. We also examine the personal costs and benefits of making the shift and provide a carefully selected, powerful set of strategies—strategies that are easy to implement and have a very high ratio of payoff to effort—for speeding your transition to effectiveness for the future.

In Chapter One, we provide the rationale and theoretical framework for the changes presented in the manager's role. We identify the changes in the health care industry that have dramatic implications for the management role. We present the "Willing and Able Matrix" as a blueprint that explains how health care managers need to respond in the face of pressure to demonstrate consistently higher levels of performance, energy, and stamina. We then summarize the ten specific role shifts required of managers who want to thrive and be valued agents of change in their organizations. Finally, we summarize the kinds of practical strategies managers can use to help them make each role shift.

Chapters Two through Eleven are devoted to the ten role shifts. The first four role shifts emphasize human resource challenges that are certainly key to management effectiveness given worker shortages, burgeoning work force diversity, and the need to upgrade employee skills constantly to keep up with customer expectations and technological change.

Chapter Two explores the need for managers to shift from a customer orientation to a provider orientation. It presents the Service Matrix as a planning device for defining customers and their service requirements, identifying strengths and weaknesses in relation to those requirements, and setting priorities for advancing customer satisfaction. It also provides a simple method of auditing the culture in your span of influence to determine the extent to which it drives service quality and continuous improvement. Finally, it includes a step-by-step plan for a staff meeting you can use to engage your staff in identifying customer needs and in problem solving to heighten customer satisfaction.

Chapter Three presents the need for a shift in attitude from getting by to raising standards. Because continuous quality improvement is increasingly a business necessity, we address the need for managers to stop tolerating marginal performance and to push standards ever upward. Strategies include how to resolve your mixed feelings about performance so that you can raise your standards and help staff move from good to great in their own behavior.

Chapter Four turns the buzzword *empowerment* into concrete management actions. It examines the need to empower employees by providing them with the tools and latitude needed to satisfy their customers. It also provides activities for helping staff develop confidence and judgment so that they will seize increasing degrees of personal responsibility.

Chapter Five reviews work force trends that affect employee attitudes and identifies key actions for managers that spark heightened employee satisfaction, loyalty, and retention. Easy-to-use techniques foster employee involvement and communicate recognition of employee contributions.

Chapters Six, Seven, and Eight address three role shifts that constitute a sorely needed bias toward action and results. In Chapter Six, we weigh the payoffs of reactive management that cause so many managers to remain reactive despite increasingly dire consequences for the organization. We then provide a series of techniques to use in preparing for and trying out a proactive approach. The "Making Your Case" technique, for example, helps you to think through an important proactive project in an efficient manner that also heightens the probability of significant results.

Chapter Seven poses the need to rethink inherited, unquestioned practices and experiment with new and better ways. It defines the experimenter mindset and provides methods for adopting fresh perspective in the face of recurrent problems. It also helps you to adjust your self-talk so that risk taking is more appealing than appalling.

In Chapter Eight, we question the value of working hard for its own sake and press instead for single-minded attention to results. We provide techniques to help you monitor results and also ask yourself and others questions that elevate the importance of results, solutions, answers, and accomplishments.

The chapters on the last three role shifts examine key management approaches consonant with heightened levels of teamwork, cohesion, and identity with your organization.

In Chapter Nine, we identify the compelling need for

management actions that make your organization "seamless," so that people, communication, and information flow smoothly across department lines. The techniques we provide are a series of meeting formats you can use with other managers to approach success levels of cooperation, teamwork, and mutual support.

In Chapter Ten, we identify management practices that have a divisive effect and propose alternative approaches that minimize finger pointing and create instead a "we feeling" and a broader perspective on the organization.

Chapter Eleven addresses the last of the ten shifts. This chapter points out the far-reaching, destructive effects of negativism in management and builds a case for choosing to reflective a positive, optimistic stance in relation to your job, your employees, and the organization. Based on the premise that optimism is a stance you have the power to adopt in the face of whatever your circumstances are, this chapter also provides techniques to help you see what is positive around you and help your employees do the same.

Finally, in Chapter Twelve, we address the reality that managers cannot successfully embrace these ambitious new role demands without some degree of executive and organizational support. Specifically, we identify the nature of the support needed from executive management in order for managers to achieve and sustain high levels of performance.

Acknowledgments

We express our gratitude and appreciation to the many people who contributed their insight, energy, and support.

The many executives and managers we worked with across the nation helped us understand their frustrations, problems, and secrets of success and also shared their frank and cogent reactions to our concepts, assertions, and strategies suggested in their formative stages.

The unceasingly energetic and supportive staff of The Einstein Consulting Group helped us address tough questions, overcome stumbling blocks, and bring this manuscript to fruition. Thank you, Susan Afriat, Amanda Blumenthal, Katie Buckley, Jack Fein, Allan Geller, Wesley Hilton, Bill Johnson, Jeanne Joseph, Beverly Mays, Gail Murphy, Jackie Riley, Loren Shuman, Joan Theetge, Sheila Wallace, Kelly Yeager, and Virginia Yeager.

The executives and managers of the Albert Einstein Healthcare Foundation, the Albert Einstein Medical Center, the Philadelphia Psychiatric Center, and the Willowcrest Bamberger Restorative Care Facility provided our firsthand grounding in management realities as well as enduring support for our consulting group in the Albert Einstein Healthcare Foundation family.

Our partners, children, sisters, brothers, parents, grandparents, colleagues, neighbors, and friends endlessly motivate us to do what we can to make the health care system provide quality care and service.

Thank you.

Philadelphia, Pennsylvania   Wendy Leebov
July 1990   Gail Scott

The Authors

Wendy Leebov is president of The Einstein Consulting Group, a subsidiary of the Albert Einstein Healthcare Foundation in Philadelphia. She received her B.A. degree (1966) from Oberlin College in sociology/anthropology. She received her Ed.M. degree (1967) and her Ed.D. degree (1971) from the Harvard Graduate School of Education in human development. With more than twenty years of experience in management development, team building, and organizational change, Leebov is a nationally recognized speaker and currently provides consulting and training services to health care organizations nationwide in the areas of service excellence, total quality improvement, and management development and renewal.

Her first book, *Service Excellence: The Customer Relations Strategy for Health Care* (1988), is widely recognized as the industry standard for service excellence strategy. Her numerous publications include her second book, *Patient Satisfaction: A Guide to Practice Enhancement* (1989, with M. Vergare and G. Scott), and articles in *Health Care Management Review, Journal of Healthcare Marketing, Hospitals,* and many other journals. She is also editor of *Service Excellence in Practice*, a bimonthly subscription newsletter.

Gail Scott is currently director of consultation and training for The Einstein Consulting Group. She received her B.A. degree (1975) and her M.A. degree (1977) from Beaver College, both in theater and English. With her team of consultants, Scott has helped more than 200 health care organizations institute far-reaching, long-term approaches to building high-performance management teams and achieving a competitive edge through service excellence. She has developed with Wendy Leebov the widely acclaimed "Service Management Essentials" and "New Vital Manager" management development programs. She is also coauthor of *Patient Satisfaction: A Guide to Practice Enhancement* (1989).

Health Care Managers
in Transition

A New Era
for Health Care Managers

Managers in health care have never had it easy. Unlike our counterparts in industry, our goals are not only growth, a sound bottom line, a well-oiled machine, or better widgets. Our overarching goal is to help people get well and to comfort and care for them in the best manner technologically and humanely possible.

Although our multiple purposes and humanitarian ideals complicate the basic management job, these very forces also inspire health care managers to the level of commitment and dedication necessary to meet complex challenges.

Although the job of health care manager has always appeared difficult, it seems far more difficult today. Today's health care industry is in perpetual motion. Rules that applied a decade ago are obsolete, and that fact affects everyone who works in health care. The pressures and anxieties imposed by competition, diminishing resources, changing reimbursement, staffing shortages, alternative delivery systems, changing relationships between hospitals and physicians, administrative turnover, multicultural work forces and patients, morale problems, and other factors have placed

1

health care organizations and their personnel in a position of uncertainty.

Obsolescence of Status Quo Management

Eight trends, not all unique to the health care industry, now challenge the relevance of "traditional" management practices and call for a dramatically new job description: (1) more demanding consumers, (2) increasing competition, (3) changing work force values, (4) new reimbursement rules that drive decision making, (5) changing requirements of the Joint Commission for the Accreditation of Healthcare Organizations (JCAHO), (6) the organizational structure shuffle, (7) the need to do more with fewer resources, and (8) new demands on top management.

More Demanding Consumers. Our customers are increasingly demanding. Health care consumers are noticeably more attuned to their health care alternatives than ever before. And they have more of them. They demand the latest technology, convenient in their communities, without compromising high-touch care. And, they view health care providers with an astutely critical eye. Suspicions about the stereotyped "greedy, disinterested physician" and the "intimidating, overpriced hospital" have caused many consumers to turn to self-care and alternative health care providers. As a result, consumers are increasingly aware of their power over health care organizations whom they see competing openly to attract their business. The consumer tests us with high expectations. And they hold us accountable to our promises. In the past, a few rude words from a health care worker would be par for the consumer's course. Now, that consumer wants not only an explanation but also, often, reparations. If we do not respond to their expectations in a satisfactory manner, consumers are likely to sue or spread the word about the organization to friends and go to St. Somewhere Else the next time they need health care.

Under the scrutinizing eye of the consumer, we have to

enable our staff to accomplish more than ever, better than our competitors, faster and more cost-effectively, and with a smile.

And when our organizations do not meet customer expectations, who is responsible? Managers—the people who run the place on the inside.

A tall order.

Increasing Competition. Competition is old hat to health care managers. Yet their personal involvement in the competitive challenge is increasing. Administrators and Boards are intensifying the pressure to win on quality, service, technology, and price, while operating lean and mean departments. Pressure to compete effectively is moving from the global level in the organization down into departments, units, and product lines. Managers at every level more often than not have escalating responsibility for increasing market share, adding value to services rendered, and helping the organization strengthen its competitive position. This active participation in the competitive race is anathema to many managers, especially the many who have moved straight from technical and clinical backgrounds into management positions.

A tall order.

Changing Work Force Values. Values are changing among health care workers, as well as other workers. Employees today tend less than before to devote themselves to their employer and give their all. They know painfully well that their employer cannot in good conscience promise them job security and steadily escalating salaries. Thus, workers expect the employer to meet more of their needs in the short run to maintain their loyalty or even their employment. According to Maccoby (1988, pp. 57–76), employees today are motivated to work by a combination of eight value drives: survival, relatedness, pleasure, information, mastery, play, dignity, and meaning.

The challenge to management is compelling. Managers need to tap employee potential in terms of output, service quality, and creativity while also meeting this demanding array of needs. The astute manager now sees each employee as a precious customer whose perseverance and loyalty are needed by the organization. One hospital CEO said it pointedly, "The manager walks a tightrope, on the one hand trying to boost output, while on the other hand taking steps to charm the employee into unquestioned dedication." It is not surprising that so many managers feel exhausted as they work hard to avoid alienating their employees while pressuring them to do more work and higher-quality work. The people management skills required to maintain this delicate balance involve sensitivity, respect, forethought, and finesse.

A tall order.

New Reimbursement Rules That Drive Decision Making. In the good old days, hospitals were reimbursed by the government and other third parties based on cost. Whatever we spent, we received in reimbursement. We had a blank check that made resource allocation and management decisions easy. No wonder we lament the good old days.

Most health care managers are already keenly aware of the fact that hospitals are (and soon physicians will be) reimbursed at the fixed rate attached to the diagnosis of the patient. If health care providers spend more than that fixed rate, they lose the difference. If they spend less, they make money.

Needless to say, this fixed rate of reimbursement (which has been steadily declining) has forced health care providers to make every second count and to eliminate waste (wasted time, wasted supplies, wasted energy). The slack is gone from what was once an infinitely elastic rope.

The impact on managers is profound. Managers are held accountable for what they do, what they spend, and the results they achieve, because these aspects of their performance have profound effects on the organization's viability in this financial squeeze. Managers have to manage on a shoestring budget and meet heightening quality standards.

A tall order.

Changing JCAHO Requirements. The process of accrediting health care organizations is also under a microscope.

Members of the JCAHO as well as health care providers agree that it is time to revamp accreditation processes to focus on "quality" as defined not only by professional standards but also by customer expectations and requirements; to emphasize "outcomes," not only "process"; and to institute quality standards for management and operations, not only clinical areas. These changes impose new pressures on health care organizations, especially on managers. The emphasis on measurable outcomes, performance standards, and management audits means not only more work, but greater accountability and the development and institution of time-consuming operational processes. Every manager must achieve positive outcomes related to quality and customer satisfaction by setting standards, monitoring performance, and continuously improving service, all while keeping employees productive, motivated, and dedicated.

A tall order.

The Organizational Structure Shuffle. The organizational structures of many health care organizations have been destabilized. Shifts to product line management, mergers, buyouts, and corporate restructuring abound. Although these structural changes can provide new opportunities, they also generate upheaval and uncertainty within the organization's walls and in the hearts and minds of its employees: What does this mean to me? Will I have a job? Will my friends leave? Will this organization make it? How will I make the changes expected of me? These and other questions plague employees and their managers. Those among us who were promoted from technical to management positions because of our technical savvy now must help employees deal with an erratic mixture of fright, insecurity, anger, worry, and indifference. Suddenly, we need to build confidence, inspire, reassure, support, and nurture employees to sustain employee performance and keep the faith.

A tall order.

The Need to Do More with Fewer Resources. Structural instability and financial constraints are not even the worst of it. Many organizations do not have adequate numbers of care-givers, including nurses, technicians, and therapists. So much attention must be devoted to attracting the quantity of professionals needed to deliver care! Hospitals, ambulatory care centers, entrepreneurial service registries, consulting firms, and nursing homes are all hustling to outdo one another in their aggressive and innovative approaches to attracting and retaining talented people. Many have even lowered experience, skill, and educational standards to attract the numbers of employees needed to "cover" the patients.

In times of staffing shortages, standards of care are at risk. Staff members are overstretched, yet managers must ensure that the necessary work is done and, at the same time, nurture the employees they have and attract new ones.

A tall order.

New Demands on Top Management. All of these changes also entail a new role for executive management. Executives are managing external relationships and, increasingly, the fragile relationships with physicians who, themselves, are reeling in the face of uninvited changes in their practice environments. Executives might have found solace and satisfaction in managing operations in the past, in scrutinizing daily processes, in watching over managers and defining their priorities. Today, they do not have the time or the information needed to stay on top of daily operations.

Managers have to take over, filling the vacuum left by executives who, appropriately, must focus their energies on the tumultuous environment and the sticky and demanding relationships with payers, venture partners, and physicians that demand their undivided attention. Managers are unaccustomed to filling that vacuum; when they do move forward, they often run up against layers of red tape that have historically impeded decision making and authoritative action on their parts. They must fill that vacuum without ruffling the feathers of senior management, who also are unaccustomed to letting go of operational authority.

A tall order.

In Sum. More to do. Less to do it with. Less money overall. Fewer talented staff. More accountability. More emphasis on results. More scrutiny by the consumer and the payer. Strained relationships among key players. A high-stress environment. Less elasticity in every part of the system. A taut rope. Unpredictability and pressure. And no way to make these factors disappear.

Response of Managers to the Squeeze

At one hospital in Detroit, three department heads vent about managing in today's environment:

> I feel like the rug's been pulled out from under me. The job I was hired to do isn't the job I'm supposed to be doing now. But frankly, I'm not really sure *what* I'm supposed to be doing now!

> This job used to be a nice, secure thing. I'd come to work every day. I'd pump up the troops. I'd make sure my department was functioning smoothly—that all bases were covered. I'd mind my own business. I'd respond to requests from my boss. When I felt overloaded, I'd just do what I could and let the other things fall through cracks. No one would really notice anyway. I'd solve problems in my department, but you couldn't do much about the bigger problems, and anyway, they'd gone on for years. To tell you the truth, I think I've done a real good job over the years. But now, I'm not so sure.

> The industry has gone berserk and I think top management is taking it out on us. They expect the impossible and they're never satisfied. It's worse than "do more with less." They're saying, "Do the impossible with nothing!"

At a large teaching hospital in Boston, managers are talking:

> I feel stuck between a rock and a hard place. My
> employees look to me to make their lives easier
> because they're under stress. And my boss keeps
> loading more work on me. *Every*thing is a prior-
> ity. I'll tell you that I'm having a very tough time
> responding to my staff's needs and my boss' end-
> less demands at the same time.

> To tell you the truth, I don't know what
> I'm supposed to be doing anymore. There's an
> atmosphere of panic and neverending work. But
> I think we're chasing our tails. No one really has
> a fix on where we're going and how we're going
> to get there.

> I'm having a great time. I was getting
> bored with my job, but lately, there's so much
> confusion and so much need for change, that you
> can get out of the rut and try new things. Before,
> the way we always did everything here was
> sacred. You couldn't change it even if it hadn't
> worked in years. Now, everything's up for grabs.
> And I'm grabbing.

At a midsized hospital in a Texas suburb, managers lament:

> Either I'm so stressed that I need medical care
> myself, or I'm so busy that I might as well move
> in here, so I can work night and day. How's my
> family taking this? That's another story.

> I don't sweat it. I'm sitting back and waiting
> it out. I've been here for 23 years. I've watched one
> whippersnapper after another try their hands at
> running this place. Every one of them says they're
> going to change the place, but not much ever really

happens. I know I'll outlast them. I always do.
There's no sense getting bothered by the pressure.
I'm just going to wait it out.

The health care environment is unlikely to stabilize in
the near future. Frankly, those people hoping for a reprieve—
awaiting the day when the pressures will ease—are kidding
themselves and setting themselves up for substantial disappointment. We have suffered at the hands of our own complacency. Now, we have to regroup and make the changes
needed to act effectively in the face of what will undoubtedly
be an ongoing barrage of unforeseen circumstances.

Today's environment demands that managers reach new
heights of accomplishment and stamina, based on a new,
empowering and invigorating mindset. To help their organizations adapt rapidly to this fluid environment, managers
must heighten their hardiness, flexibility, adaptability, resilience, leadership, and stamina to embrace the challenges now
inherent in the job.

"Middle management . . . is an obsolete profession, at
least in its present form," according to Deal and Kennedy
(1982, p. 186). To spur the far-reaching changes needed in the
role of health care manager, nothing short of a paradigm
shift is needed. Lawler (1987) describes the core paradigm
shift as that from "control" to "commitment/involvement."

At the heart of the traditional "control" model is the
quest to establish order, assert control, and realize efficiency
in the way employees perform their jobs. The control model
is most often reflected in the following organizational norms
(Bradford and Cohen, 1984):

• The good manager knows at all times what is going on
  in the department.
• The good manager should have more technical expertise
  than any subordinate.
• The good manager should be able to solve any problems
  that come up (or at least solve the problem before the
  subordinate).

- The good manager should be the primary (if not the only) person responsible for how the department is functioning.

Also, according to Bellman (1988), managers grounded in the control model make decisions based on established directions; emphasize the rational; use given resources effectively; work according to plans and schedules; are analytical, objective, and practical; act in the present, based on the past; and emphasize knowledge and facts. Although this model has always had some problems, these days, its negative consequences are blatant and far-reaching. Turbulence, as an industry "given," does not fit comfortably into the control mentality. Because the only constant is change, we cannot prescribe every role, define every position, maintain inelastic accountability standards, all typical and necessary components of the control paradigm. The linear approach to management typical of the control model proceeds from mission to goals to strategies to objectives to plans to business units. But with change so rapid, by the time we complete this procession, we would find ourselves implementing what made sense yesterday, not today. In the bureaucracies of the past, change at a snail's pace was the best we could do, but this does not work now when we need to expedite a steady stream of changes for the sake of survival and improved quality of care. We need a paradigm that triggers quicker starts and stops, more experimentation, and responsiveness to the environment—a more flexible paradigm.

Changes in the work force further tax the control model. Neither deference to authority nor unquestioned loyalty to the employer can be expected. Employees want more influence over a whole host of issues—procedures, schedules, incentives, hiring, organizational policy, and so on (Lawler, Renwick, and Bullock, 1981).

What is the alternative to the control model? The commitment/involvement paradigm for the management role invokes broader responsibility with greater employee involvement in decisions; adaptability; individual initiative to constantly upgrade practices, policies, performance, and results;

open communication; and interdependency and integration among organizational units via managerial actions. To these, Bellman (1988) adds decision making based on a vision of the future; action based on intuition and supported by reason; expansion beyond given resources; work based on what is needed now, not on rigid plans and schedules; a vision of the future based on the present, not the past; and an emphasis on belief and commitment, not only knowledge and facts.

Managers who want to thrive, earn support and respect as leaders, and achieve results important to the organization's mission and longevity must change their mindsets and behavior in line with this basic paradigm shift.

It is nothing short of a new job.
No rules. No map. No wonder.

To better define the nature of this essential transformation, in this book we define and explore in some depth ten role shifts managers need to make, shifts that reposition the manager for effectiveness within the commitment/involvement paradigm.

Ten Role Shifts

From	To
Provider orientation	Customer orientation
Getting by	Raising standards
Director	Empowerer
Employee as expendable resource	Employee as customer
Reactive behavior	Proactive behavior
Tradition and safety	Experimentation and risk
Busyness	Results
Turf protection	Teamwork across lines
"We-they" thinking	Organizational perspective
Cynicism	New optimism

This sounds like rhetoric until you try to exemplify the new role requirements. It is not easy to make these shifts if your organization reinforced "the old way."

Some executive teams and some health care cultures are ready for managers to function in new ways and encourage their managers through word *and* deed to make the necessary transitions. In other organizations, however, managers who want to be full contributors and set the pace for progress encounter obstacle after obstacle, regardless of the executive team's rhetoric. Then, when these managers do what executives claim to want, they find themselves paying negative consequences. Your ability to be successful in your role depends partly on the people, policies, practices, and incentives that constitute your environment.

In Chapter Twelve, we will identify the organizational supports you need to sustain performance in line with new role demands, and identify steps you can take to secure this needed support.

When you see a list like the ten role shifts, the temptation is to interpret the shifts as from "bad" to "good." Resist this temptation, because such an interpretation can lead to inappropriate judgments about yourself and other managers who may have performed in a style appropriate to the past.

The point is that the approaches on the left, now considered the old way, did work. The managers who operated accordingly felt effective. These methods do not work today because the environment and its requirements have changed. At one time, employees felt secure in their jobs and loyal to the organization. Now, job security is not a given, and managers must seek different motivators to foster dedication among their staff. At one time, managers had barely any unwelcome news—for example, layoffs, freezes, downsizing, lack of funds to replace broken equipment, and turnover—to communicate to employees. Now, managers need to communicate this news more often and in such a way that employees keep their faith in the organization. At one time, performance of the organization, its managers, and departments was considered adequate. Now, in the face of resource constraints, competition, and rising quality standards, new solutions must be found for longstanding problems.

These demands and many more are the product of

changing times and industry trends. Effective managers of the past will continue to be effective only if they change to meet the new demands.

Some managers are stimulated by the changing environment and these new role demands; others are buckling under to the new pressures and expectations.

In the face of new role demands and pressures, managers vary on two critical dimensions: their willingness to embrace new role demands and their ability to do what is needed to meet these demands with skill and efficiency (Figure 1). Some managers are "willing and able." They are open to meeting the new demands and they energetically expand their repertoires and responsibilities so they can manage competently in the new environment.

Other managers are "willing and unable." Intent on doing all they can to move the organization forward, they are open to making the needed role changes, but feel inadequate to the task. The new role demands call for skills in marketing, quality assurance, cost containment, forecasting, systems and product design, innovation, motivation, and much more—skills that fall beyond their comfort and competence zones.

Still other managers are "unwilling and able." They

Figure 1. The Willing and Able Matrix.

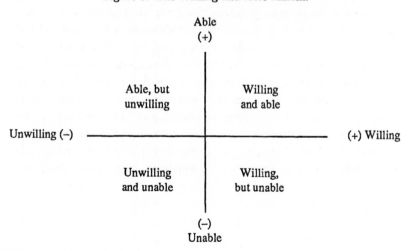

already have or they know how to develop needed skills, but they resist. They have become comfortable with their management role as is and do not want to make the changes asked of them. Some resent the pressure to change and resist, believing that they will outlast the administrators making the new demands on them. Others expect or hope that the environment will change, or believe that their ways are the right ways, making role changes premature and misguided.

Still other managers are "unwilling and unable." They lack the skills they need to meet the new demands and, on top of that, they resist role changes with what often appears to others as stubbornness and rigidity.

The value placed on membership in the four categories just described is dramatically changing. In the past, willing and able managers were often labeled derogatorily as "mavericks" and were subtly expelled from the organization because of their determination to make change, to try new ways, and to question outmoded traditions. The able, but unwilling managers were the "in group." If you joined them at lunch, you could count on vigorous griping, finger pointing, and cynicism about an astounding variety of obstacles, problems, bosses, and personalities—all of which, they claimed, made it impossible to accomplish much on the job. A warm camaraderie often developed within this group, with outsiders feeling somehow naive and prudish.

If we were to attach names to the groups on the basis of their social value and role within the culture in the past, the matrix might look like that in Figure 2.

To gain acceptance and comfort within the organization, some mavericks made the changes necessary to "fit" better into the culture, squelching their experimental nature so they could gain admission to the in group. The result was status quo management.

But no more. Today, the social value ascribed to managers in the four categories is changing. As the organization can no longer survive with status quo management, the benefits reaped from unwillingness and inability are dwindling. As more managers move to the ranks of the willing and able,

Figure 2. The Willing and Able Matrix of the Past.

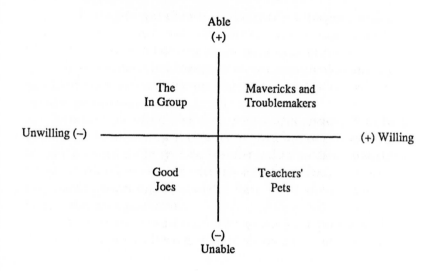

Figure 3. The Willing and Able Matrix Redefined.

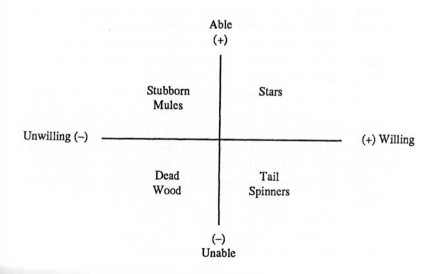

the in group is being redefined with the strong urging of visionary executives who know what it will take to move their organizations through the rapids of change.

The evolving status associated with membership in each of the four categories is illustrated in Figure 3. The able, but unwilling manager, once comfortable in the in group, is now viewed as a stubborn mule who resists inevitable and important changes. The willing, but unable managers were once the favorite of many executive teams because of their unflinching team player attitude and loyalty. Now they are viewed as tail spinners who work hard, but do not reap the results the organization requires. The good Joes, who constituted the unwilling and unable category, are now openly referred to as deadwood. And the willing and able managers, once looked at askance as mavericks, even troublemakers, have become the shining stars.

The question is, What will my organization require from its managers and how can I reposition myself to help the organization adapt in response to change?

Organizations need willing and able managers. Only willing and able managers can mobilize the talent and energy that have become business necessities. Only willing and able managers can accept this new era as a time of adventure and motivate themselves and co-workers to seize the inherent opportunities with a positive mindset. Unwilling and unable managers drag themselves, their people, and their organizations down.

Repositioning

If you have assessed your own position relative to the ten role shifts examined here and find that you need to change, you can reposition yourself if you are determined to do so. To help, we offer a variety of recommendations grounded in five premises.

Premise 1: Your belief system and the way you conceptualize your management role, that is, your "mindset," powerfully influence your managerial behavior and effectiveness. The lens you wear shapes what you see and do. For example, if you look at your organization through suspicious or cynical "glasses," you will mistrust your executive team and constantly look over your shoulder for signs of threat or oppression. If, on the other hand, you wear trusting glasses, you will see your executive team as supportive. Mindset shapes and drives behavior and priorities.

Therefore, it is efficient in terms of your time and energy to rethink whether you have the management mindset you want and, if not, to change it so that your behavior will fall in line accordingly. You can thus change many behavioral patterns at one time, rather than one at a time.

Premise 2: The role shifts we describe involve a continuum of thought and action. It is not black and white. Although some people behave rigidly, many more people are flexible and capable of moving from one point to another along a continuum depending on the situation. For example, regarding the continuum from turf protection to teamwork, you might cross turf lines easily to join a colleague on an exciting innovative project, but remain territorial and secretive with respect to competition for scarce budgetary resources. You can move along the continuum in the direction you choose, one step at a time. Eventually, your prevalent style, or modus operandi, will shift to conform more spontaneously and consistently to the new role demands.

Premise 3: Performance at each end of the continuum has costs and benefits, for you personally and for the organization. This makes the decision to change difficult because you may lose something of personal value by changing. You would not be managing the way you are if you did not reap benefits. So, when faced with pressure to change, you stand to lose those benefits associated with your current style of management. Although we hope to convince you that repositioning is adaptive and necessary and has benefits too, you may still resist. Because your organization needs you to change whether you want to or not, become aware of the costs and benefits of changing versus not changing, so you can at least grapple frontally with your resistance to change and the difficulty that change creates for you. Managers who do not stop to consider what they are gaining from their current patterns of thought and action run the risk of making a lip-service commitment to change because it is trendy to do so, while they inwardly resist real change tenaciously.

Premise 4: You can change your own mindset if you choose to. You have that power. We posit that you have the power to decide how your job should be done. You can control your own thoughts and actions if you want to. If you work in a culture that mitigates against the mindset shifts we propose, you can decide to go with the flow of the traditional culture. Or, you can act differently and help to reshape that culture. You have the power to think and act in whichever way you choose, knowing of course that each way has consequences for you and the organization.

Premise 5: If you do decide to change your mindset, you can ease your journey by experimenting with your actions and your thoughts. Consider this triangle:

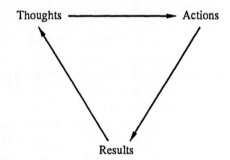

Your thoughts, your actions, and your results affect each other. If you think "customers come first," you are likely to act calmly and responsively in the face of a patient complaint. On the other hand, if you think "I come first," you are more likely to resent the patient for interfering with your peace of mind. In other words, what you think to yourself about yourself and the situation at hand affects your actions.

Now, consider our claim that your actions affect your

results. If you think "customers come first" and then react calmly and responsively to a complaint, the patient will probably feel better about both you and the organization. If, however, you think "me first" and express your annoyance in an abrupt and defensive response, the patient will be offended and think poorly of you and the organization.

The results you obtain in the many situations you face constitute experience that reinforces your thoughts and, in turn, affects subsequent action, in a cyclical fashion.

If you choose to change to meet new role demands, you can ease your journey by intervening at either of two entry points: your thoughts or your actions.

In the following chapters, we present strategies to help you decide to alter your thoughts or your actions. Specifically, we make explicit the type of thinking that weds managers to old-style management. We identify a different way of thinking that characterizes managers who have made the transition to meet today's requirements.

If you prefer to alter or strengthen your position along the continuum by altering your actions first (which will, in turn, affect your thoughts and results), we provide behavioral strategies. By acting differently, you will achieve different results, which will reinforce different thoughts and thereby reinforce your new role.

The changes outlined here may upset you or provide you with an adventure, depending on your world view at this time. Peters (1987) claims that middle management ranks will slim by 80 percent over the next few years, leaving only 20 percent of us in middle management jobs. If you want to be among the 20 percent who survive and, better yet, thrive, then you must reposition yourself to be effective in our changing environment. Managers who perpetually renew and reeducate themselves and willingly make the necessary changes have the best chance of surviving the turbulence.

If you rise to the occasion, you will not feel bored or stuck in your job. Rising to meet new role demands means challenge, stretch, development, and new possibilities for those who choose to do so with energy and alacrity.

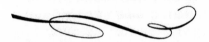

From a Provider
to a Customer Orientation

1. Do you decide to use systems and procedures purely on the basis of staff convenience and ease of use? YES NO
2. Do you think you are the best judge of how well your department or division is doing? YES NO
3. Do you orient new employees only on the technical aspects of their jobs, because the rest is common sense? YES NO
4. Do you resist a customer focus because customers have unrealistic expectations and you can never satisfy them? YES NO
5. With respect to customer complaints, do you believe that "No news is good news"? YES NO
6. Do you routinely verbalize your commitment to excellent customer service to your employees? YES NO
7. Are you and your employees clear about who your customers are, both internally and externally? YES NO

8. Do you have in place methods to measure customer satisfaction?   YES NO
9. Do you celebrate successful customer satisfaction with your staff?   YES NO
10. When faced with different ways to do things, do you decide on the basis of what would be best for your customers?   YES NO

A "yes" to any of the first five questions and a "no" to the last five questions indicate a "provider orientation." If your answers reflect this orientation, do not be disheartened. Historically, many health care managers have been provider oriented, not customer oriented, for very good reasons. Until the eighties, managers were not expected to differentiate and cater to customers. In fact, the word *customer* was taboo in health care. The manager's job was primarily to please the boss, that is, follow the boss's directives. Managing your department or division meant keeping schedules tight, ensuring adequate staffing, and running your domain within a reasonable, although flexible budget. Outside pressures were few and internal competition was rare. Your role was relatively clear.

The following diagram depicts the power hierarchy that existed until very recently. The role of each group was to cater to the needs and expectations of the group above it.

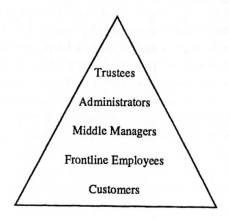

Today, the most important group in every service industry is the customer. And hospitals have only now realized that is what they are—service organizations. Customers now prevail. The pyramid must be turned upside down.

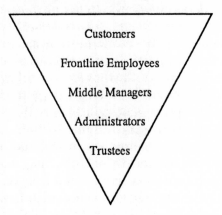

Customers

Frontline Employees

Middle Managers

Administrators

Trustees

Each group still caters to the needs and expectations of the group above it, but everyone's job has changed. Frontline employees focus on pleasing patients and their families. The job of the frontline supervisor is to make this possible. Your function as manager is to ensure that your staff have the skills and resources they need to satisfy patients and their families or those co-workers in other departments who serve patients and their families. Your success depends on keeping the customer clearly in mind and running your domain accordingly.

The preceding describes a departure from a provider orientation. Managers with a provider orientation:

• View the need to focus on customer requirements as "one more added pressure." Especially in the hospital environment, where the needs of physicians, employees, trustees, administrators, and patients often conflict, it is much easier to base decisions on one's own, not the customer's, perspective.

• Believe you cannot please everyone, so why bother.

- Think that because the system has worked so far, it should not be changed.
- Feel that it is easier to get others to adjust to them (their departments) than to adjust their practices to so many different groups. That is, the attention on customer needs creates impossible demands that cannot be met.
- Create systems, schedules, and policies without consulting the customer.
- See educating customers to "our way" as a means of gaining satisfaction and confidence.

Managers with a customer orientation:

- Focus on satisfying customers to the best of their ability.
- Define who their customers are, both internally and externally, and extensively research what customers want and expect.
- Measure success by customer satisfaction.
- Make important management decisions on the basis of their implications for customer satisfaction.
- Find out how customers perceive the services delivered.
- Repeatedly communicate the importance of a customer orientation to staff with conviction.
- Screen job applicants for both technical competence and customer interaction skills.

In the following situations, consider the differences in approach between a provider and a customer orientation.

Case 1: All of the non–revenue-generating departments, including yours, have been hit with budget cuts this year. All of your customers are internal. You know that you must reduce staff and the amount of service you provide to other departments. You must determine the basis on which you will make the cutbacks. Managers with a provider orientation ask, What can I eliminate that will wreak the least havoc with my people? Who can I live without? They make these crucial decisions based on what is easiest, with little customer consciousness or staff input. Managers with a provider orientation expect others to adjust, adapt, and accept them.

On the other hand, managers with a customer orientation approach this situation quite differently. They recognize that any cuts in service will have an impact on the ability of other departments to deliver service to patients. Recognizing that the job is to provide quality support to these departments, these managers actively solicit input from others to determine which services would be affected most severely by cuts. Customer-oriented managers evaluate the options with customer satisfaction as a central criterion, and sometimes must make very painful staffing decisions as a result.

Case 2: Physicians have been complaining about the poor service extended by your department. Your administrator has said, "Keep the docs happy!" Some provider-oriented managers may believe that there is no way to satisfy these physicians. They simply are too demanding. These managers voice a litany of excuses for failure to resolve or avoid these complaints. Other provider-oriented managers may approach these physicians personally, offering them the same excuses and blaming other people for the problems the physicians encountered. This approach is meant to "stop the complaints at any cost."

Customer-oriented managers, however, become personally involved and search for the root of the problem. Even if the physicians are notorious complainers, these managers investigate their complaints and take steps to avoid the conditions that led to these complaints.

Case 3: Your hospital is implementing a customer hotline to handle problems and complaints. The department managing this new hotline expects managers throughout the organization to handle patient, physician, or family problems related to their specific areas. Hotline staff log calls and track problems. The intention is to handle all problems immediately and to identify recurring problems that warrant preventive problem solving. You need to prepare to do your part in this system. Provider-oriented managers see this as one more headache. They are concerned about being called after hours and having to solve problems that are only marginally their responsibility. On the other hand, customer-oriented managers are excited about the new system. They recognize that many problems fall through the cracks and patients lose out as a result. They also know how difficult it is to stay on top of operations from a customer point of view, but view the new system as a help. Customer-oriented managers know that if they are not aware of a problem, they cannot fix it. They see fixing systems and solving problems as making life easier for customers in the long run and that is what matters.

Case 4: During strategy planning, the administrative team considers various clinical programs it may strengthen to make them "centers of excellence" that attract patients. A provider-oriented administrative team might ask, Which doctors would we most like to promote because they are easier to work with? And in which areas do we already have quality people and equipment? The customer-oriented administrative team looks first at community needs and customer expectations. Its decision to invest in one area over another is driven by customer needs, not its own convenience and preferences.

The difference in approach between the provider-oriented and the customer-oriented manager is profound. It is a difference in mindset—an understanding that priorities must be defined by customer, not personal, needs. The customer must be foremost.

The Strains Inherent in a Customer Orientation

Many managers have not welcomed what was once an invitation and is now pressure to shift to a customer orientation. If you are the least bit resistant to adopting a customer orientation, do not feel alone. Managers we have listened to admit that the provider orientation remains appealing. Some talk about the many people you have to please if you are customer oriented, people you do not have to please when you are inattentive to customers' special wants and needs. The provider-oriented manager does not allow exceptions or make changes in routine procedures and does not have to confront staff problems, because he or she is insulated from customer feedback.

Even if you are determined to adopt a customer orientation, the transition is not at all simple. Many systems need to be revamped once you make the customer central. If you have not been schooled in a customer consciousness and service management technique, the tools needed will not be handy. Some managers feel they must negate all they have learned in the past and start over with neither role models nor supportive management systems and leadership. Although we can learn from those other industries that are ahead of us in customer orientation (for example, airlines and hotels), health care organizations are much more complex and the analogy is therefore strained. The vulnerability of our patients, differing acuity levels, complex, rapidly changing technology, and the high degree of specialization necessary make our jobs that much harder.

Some managers and many frontline professionals reject the emphasis on customer service, believing that our job is to make people well using our expertise. We are the experts and we know what is best. That is the essence of the job, not customer service! So what if patients need to wait? What if they do not have a current magazine to make the time go faster? What if we keep a customer on hold several minutes? In the light of what we [health care workers] have to deal with, they should accept this.

Benefits of a Customer Orientation

On the other hand, managers who have successfully made the transition have good things to say:

> If you listen to customers and change your ways based on what they say, you make things run more smoothly. Staff are less hassled, you have fewer hassles with customers, and you don't get so many complaints.

I feel more challenged, because when customers call the shots and I listen, there are new challenges every day.

I feel vital. People who resist the power of the customer are stuck in the dark ages.

I feel better about my contribution and so does my staff *and* my boss. After all, we are a service industry and if we aren't serving our customers well, what are we in it for? Pride comes from going the extra mile for customers.

The job is really much more creative, because you're always trying to give customers solutions, added value, or something intangible that your competition can't give. It's a tremendous challenge.

Although there are some disadvantages to a customer orientation and many payoffs to a provider orientation, you limit your own options if you shun the need to shift. Competitive organizations cannot afford to allow their managers the latitude to resist much longer. Patients and physicians are more knowledgeable and demand better-quality service. They are increasingly aware of alternative providers and shop largely on the basis of service. The competitive hospital is the hospital with customer-oriented managers. Managers who are not customer driven must make the change, and fast, or they risk being a casualty of "flattened management ranks."

Strategies for Strengthening Your Customer Orientation

To expedite your transition to a customer orientation, we offer four pivotal strategies: (1) Gain perspective by viewing your service through the customer's eyes; (2) Strengthen your culture to support customer satisfaction; (3) Follow the path of continuous service improvement; and (4) Reinforce the service consciousness among your employees by allotting time for valuable staff meetings.

Strategy 1: Gain perspective by viewing your service through the customer's eyes. To entertain the true importance of what seems like an unnecessary expenditure of time to so many managers, try this brief exercise:

Step 1   Close your eyes.
Step 2   Before you read further, cover or remove your watch so you cannot see it. Do not look at it.
Step 3   Now, from memory, draw your watch. Do your best to accurately record every detail on the face of your watch.
Step 4   Now, compare your watch with your drawing.
Step 5   Count the number of details you missed or drew incorrectly.

What is the point? Very few people can accurately draw their own watch. Most people miss about five key details: they draw second hands and numbers where there were none; they incorrectly represent or omit the color, brand name, and shape; and they omit other items present on the face. Yet most of us look at our watch dozens of times in the course of a day. Would you not expect, then, to be completely familiar with every detail? Do you not assume that you know your watch as well as, say, the back of your hand?

You may know your watch so well that you take it for granted. You do not notice the details anymore. You see only what you need to see.

The same is true of your work group and services. You see the same people, behaving the same way, providing the same services, using the same procedures every day. One manager of a busy emergency department told us how shocked she was to be told by outsiders that two chairs were broken in the waiting room, that two-year-old notices were still posted on the bulletin board, that the toilet seat was cracked, that holiday decorations were hanging in the waiting room (in

June), and, finally, that the chief resident was not only chewing gum but also blowing bubbles while examining patients. All this was news to her, even though she "saw" it everyday.

How can you keep your perspective when your environment becomes so familiar? You must solicit feedback from your internal and external customers. You need their fresh eyes.

One helpful guide to soliciting customer feedback is the Service Matrix (Figure 4) developed by The Einstein Consulting Group (1985). On the left side, the Service Matrix delineates five key components of service excellence, components that affect the satisfaction of the various customers served by an organization.

You can use the Service Matrix to expand your perspective by asking members of each customer group to give you feedback on the five service components, that is, their requirements and their perceptions of your current strengths and weaknesses.

There are several ways to solicit feedback, including focus groups, surveys, and interviews. There now follows a step-by-step guide to conducting a customer focus group, a particularly effective way to obtain rich, qualitative feedback from your customers.

A focus group is a small discussion group organized to learn others' view of your service. A facilitator is needed to guide the discussion using a question guide. Focus groups work best when questions are open ended and the facilitator encourages substantial discussion of each question within the group.

To use focus groups to identify your customers' current perceptions of your service and expectations, convene representatives of only one of your customer groups at a time. One focus group might involve doctors; another, patients; and another, an internal department with which your people interact daily. The ideal focus group involves five to twelve people and lasts ninety minutes.

A staff member who is a good listener and is considered open minded, fair, and good with people should be the facilitator. It would be helpful if this person has had experience

Figure 4. The Service Matrix.

Customer Groups

Key Components	Patients	Family Friends	Physicians	Internal Customers	Group Buyers	JCAHO
Technical/Clinical Competence						
Environment						
People Skills						
Systems						
Amenities						

in leading group discussions and is able to withhold his or her own opinions and encourage communication among group members. Or your organization may employ training professionals, organization development specialists, or marketing specialists who can conduct focus groups.

The facilitator should state the purpose of the group, for example:

The engineering department is working to improve the quality of service it extends to its customers (physicians, housekeepers, and so on). You have been identified as key customers of this department. I have been asked to convene this group of [customer group] to learn what you expect from this department in the way of service, so people in the department can focus their efforts at improvement on what matters to you, their customers.

The facilitator should then introduce herself or himself and ask the members of the group to do the same.

The next step is to establish ground rules, as in this example:

Let me explain how this discussion will work. I have some questions I want you to address. I would like you to speak up and share your views. Each person in the group should answer each question. If you have something else to say, or you want to comment on what someone else said, that is great. Feel free to agree or disagree with one another. There is no need to make decisions or reach agreement. I only want to hear what you think.

I will keep what you say as an individual *confidential.* I will report only on main points and patterns. I ask you also to keep what is said here confidential, so people can feel free to speak up. Do you agree? [Wait for responses.] I will

tape-record [or take notes on] what is said, so I
do not forget it. The group will last ninety minutes. I thank you in advance for participating.

The facilitator should begin the discussion by asking
those convened what they like about the services provided
and what problems they see in the delivery of service. Now
the Service Matrix can be used to push for more specifics.
After handing out copies of the matrix or drawing it on a
flipchart or chalkboard, the facilitator should explain it, and
then probe for strengths and weaknesses in each box relevant
to the department's area of responsibility.

Facilitators, take note of the following: Throughout,
use reflective listening and paraphrasing to make sure that
you have grasped what people are saying. After one person
answers, invite other responses with cues such as, How do
other people see this? or To what extent do people agree with
that? or Does anyone see this differently? Also, be positive
and accepting (for example, say "uh-huh" and "yes?" and
nod) to encourage people to express themselves. Probe and
push, but at no time disagree with what someone says.
Express your appreciation to people for participating. Reiterate the purpose of the group, redirecting any diversions, for
example: As I said, we convened this group so we could learn
what matters to you in terms of service. We will take what we
have learned today and use it to build on the strengths and
tackle the weaknesses.

*Strategy 2: Strengthen your culture to support customer
satisfaction.* Think about the climate and culture of your
department or division. Is it supportive of great service to
customers? What systems, procedures, and strategies are in
place to create an environment that promotes customer-oriented action on the part of staff? Perhaps you take time at
staff meetings to read thank-you notes from happy customers.
Maybe you have started an employee-of-the-quarter program
or appointed a different employee each week to act as physician liaison. You and your supervisors may have initiated a
departmental newsletter on service problems and improve-

ments. Such actions help to develop a "service culture," a culture that supports customer satisfaction by making service initiative and continuous service improvement a core activity.

Leebov (1988) identifies ten forces in departmental/organizational culture that affect service quality and consequently customer satisfaction—the ten pillars of service excellence: (1) management philosophy and commitment, (2) accountability, (3) input and evaluation, (4) problem solving and complaint management, (5) systems for communication, (6) staff development and training, (7) physician involvement, (8) reward and recognition, (9) treatment of employee as customer, and (10) reminders and refreshers.

Each pillar must strongly reinforce customer orientation. Therein lies a powerful strategy for strengthening your customer orientation. Diagnose the service culture under your influence and devise ways to strengthen it.

Use the Service Culture Audit (Exhibit 1) to help you identify areas of strength and weakness in your particular department.

Exhibit 1. Service Culture Audit.

Pillar 1: Management Philosophy and Commitment

A. I actively seek resources needed to enhance customer satisfaction. YES NO
B. I actively advance our priority on customer satisfaction by allocating significant time to service improvements. YES NO
C. I routinely talk about service excellence and its importance to our work group's commitment to customers. YES NO
D. I demonstrate courtesy, concern, and responsiveness in my behavior toward customers and employees and thus serve as a positive role model. YES NO

Pillar 2: Accountability

A. Courteous, respectful, and compassionate behavior toward customers and co-workers is a requirement, not an option. YES NO
B. Employees have seen written descriptions of the service behaviors expected of them in their particular jobs. YES NO
C. Employees receive coaching and discipline, and they are terminated when they fail to meet service standards. YES NO
D. New employees are oriented to our commitment to customers and the service behaviors expected of them. YES NO

Exhibit 1. Service Culture Audit, Cont'd.

Pillar 3: Input and Evaluation

A. We seek feedback on how other departments (our internal customers) perceive our service. YES NO

B. We regularly survey our key customer groups with respect to service dimensions. YES NO

C. Employees are regularly invited to give their input on service problems and solutions. YES NO

D. We have methods for comparing service quality from one month to another. YES NO

Pillar 4: Problem Solving and Complaint Management

A. There is in place a smooth-running system for handling customer complaints. YES NO

B. Time and energy are devoted to continuous improvement of service. YES NO

C. We seek reactions from customers, including employees, to improvements we plan as a result of their complaints or requests. YES NO

D. I cross department lines to solve service problems and encourage others in my area to do so too. YES NO

Pillar 5: Systems for Communication

A. I tell and encourage others in my area to tell employees the truth when high-level decisions are made that affect their jobs. YES NO

B. Employees are regularly informed about the financial situation and what is being done to succeed. YES NO

C. Customer feedback is regularly shared with employees. YES NO

D. A variety of methods (oral and written) are used to communicate with employees. YES NO

Pillar 6: Staff Development and Training

A. People who excel at service are involved in helping others sharpen their service skills. YES NO

B. Staff are actively encouraged to take advantage of training opportunities related to heightening customer satisfaction. YES NO

C. I ensure that at least quarterly, someone conducts skill-building sessions that will help staff satisfy our customers. YES NO

D. When new people are hired, I include in their orientation meaningful coaching on job-specific opportunities to heighten customer satisfaction. YES NO

Exhibit 1. Service Culture Audit, Cont'd.

Pillar 7: Physician Involvement

A. Physicians who come in contact with my area are aware of our priority on excellent service to customers. YES NO

B. Physicians are routinely asked how we can improve delivery of our services to them. YES NO

C. A physician who violates our service standards is confronted in a constructive manner. YES NO

D. The steps necessary to build cooperative team relationships with our physicians are actively taken. YES NO

Pillar 8: Reward and Recognition

A. Employees who are courteous and helpful to customers are recognized regularly. YES NO

B. Employees value our reward and recognition efforts. YES NO

C. I ensure that staff receive frequent "pats on the back" for positive service performance. YES NO

D. Staff contributions to customer satisfaction are acknowledged. YES NO

Pillar 9: Treatment of Employee as Customer

A. I and other supervisors in my area solicit and listen to employee concerns. YES NO

B. Employees participate in planning for changes that will affect them. YES NO

C. Employees have the tools they need to serve our customers without frustration. YES NO

D. The work atmosphere is comfortable for employees. YES NO

Pillar 10: Reminders and Refreshers

A. Accomplishments and improvements that contribute to customer satisfaction are publicized. YES NO

B. Special events, for example, contests, are conducted to energize staff with respect to customer satisfaction. YES NO

C. Visual reminders of the importance of customer satisfaction can be found in our area. YES NO

D. Employees are provided feedback from customers so they can take steps to heighten satisfaction. YES NO

If you answered "no" to any item, remedy the deficiencies and strengthen the extent to which your culture heightens customer consciousness on the part of staff.

Strategy 3: Follow the path of continuous service improvement. Now that you have considered your culture and assessed your service from your customer's point of view, you need to institute a cyclical service management process, a process that enables you to monitor service quality and use your findings to continuously improve service.

The Service Quality Improvement Process (Figure 5) developed by The Einstein Consulting Group (1989) is a guide to customer-oriented management. It outlines what is needed to make conformance to customer requirements an ongoing process that fosters continuous improvement in service quality. The cyclical process illustrated in Figure 5 resembles the traditional quality improvement process, but it starts with identification of customer requirements and sparks improvements in the quality of service, not only the quality of clinical care.

Strategy 4: Reinforce the service consciousness among your employees by allotting time for valuable staff meetings. This fourth strategy instills a customer orientation within your staff, so that they work with you, not against you, as you foster the transition to customer orientation. In addition to devoting time to interactions with your staff on budgets, schedules, and projects, you need to direct some of your staff's undivided attention to the importance of customer needs.

Here is one staff meeting agenda that accomplishes this purpose—Staff Alert.

Staff Alert: A Meeting Agenda.

1. Describe your priority on service excellence and customer satisfaction.
2. Warn your employees that you will be focusing, and you want them to focus, on ways the department can become more attuned to customer needs and better able to meet or exceed them.
3. Involve employees in identifying their key customers.
4. Invite employees to evaluate the department or division on service dimensions, using the Service Matrix.

Figure 5. The Service Quality Improvement Process.

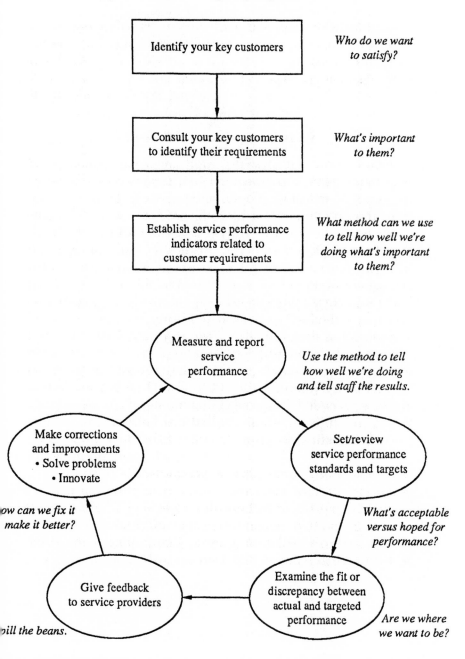

5. Describe any plans you have for launching a deliberate service improvement strategy, including perhaps formation of a service steering committee of interested staff. Solicit staff reactions to your plans and their suggestions.
6. Commit yourself to a mechanism for ongoing communication regarding customer concerns and perceptions, for example, reporting to employees the results of customer feedback, service improvement plans, and recurrent complaints.

The following outline of a meeting segment exemplifies how staff can be involved in meetings that heighten their consciousness and move them toward constructive service improvement initiatives:

*   Discuss the importance of knowing who our customers are so that we can provide the kind of service that satisfies their needs.
*   Ask employees to brainstorm their main customer groups (both internal and external).
*   Emphasize that each customer group has its own needs and expectations regarding service.
*   Divide your staff into groups of three. Ask each small group to brainstorm the expectations of customer groups.
*   Convene the whole group and compile one grand list for each customer group. One Staff Alert meeting produced the following results:

Pharmacy Department

Customer Group	Service Requirements
Patients	Quick service
	Easy-to-read instructions
	Accurate prescriptions
Nurses	Quick cooperation
	Clear labeling
	Timely delivery

Doctors	Complete information
	Courteous interactions
	Fast response

- Ask the members of the group to point out, on the basis of customer expectations, the strengths and weaknesses of the department/division and the actions necessary to heighten customer satisfaction.

A customer orientation eventually must translate into service management practices—measurement, performance tracking, problem solving, complaint prevention, accountability, and so on. These skills take time to learn. In the meantime, by forcing yourself to view service from your customers' perspective, by instituting a cyclical process for service quality improvement, and by engaging your staff in ongoing service improvements, you can advance in the desired direction.

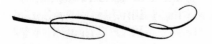

From Getting By
to Raising Standards

1. Do you believe that excellence is impossible today given staffing shortages and scarce resources?   YES NO
2. Do you believe that customer demands are becoming more and more unrealistic?   YES NO
3. Do you avoid confronting employees even when you know you should?   YES NO
4. Do you think that most people are doing a decent job?   YES NO
5. Do you believe that when it comes to excellence, people have it or do not?   YES NO
6. Do you believe that negative people should not be permitted to bring down the entire group?   YES NO
7. Do you often communicate a desire that employees stretch toward excellence, your vision of excellence?   YES NO
8. Do you exemplify excellence in your own interactions with customers and employees?   YES NO

9. Do you set and communicate ambitious performance expectations to all employees?   YES NO
10. Do you monitor employee performance on a regular basis and intervene when you see substandard behavior?   YES NO

"No" answers to the first five questions and "yes" answers to the last five questions typify managers with high standards. "Yes" answers to the first five questions and "no" answers to the last five questions characterize managers who are satisfied to simply get by.

Does Tolerance Equal Caring?

How many managers have praised, let alone tolerated employees who express remorse when confronted about having generated patient complaints? Consider Gloria, an employee who has been allowed to remain on staff even though significant facets of her performance are offensive to the organization's customers. Her boss Ralph, steeped in a culture of tolerance, kindness, and generosity, confronts Gloria occasionally, but accepts excuses for her performance. He even makes excuses for her performance and for his own reluctance to insist on improved behavior: "Nobody's perfect!" "But she's such a great typist!" "She has such serious family problems that I can't pressure her just now." Ralph, supported by the organizational culture, does not expect excellent performance from Gloria or his other employees. In fact, he tolerates so much substandard behavior, the observer wonders whether the hospital is a halfway house for difficult, poorly functioning employees rather than an organization devoted to helping patients thrive.

In today's environment, low standards just do not work. From a customer orientation, managers have to reexamine their standards and commit themselves to setting and enforcing high standards for staff performance. Without such standards, the organization's promise to deliver excellent service is a pipe dream. Also, talented staff become demoralized as

they are asked to do their own work as well as that of their
less effective peers because their bosses trust and rely on them.
They know that their less effective colleagues are hurting the
department's image, even though they receive the same pay
and benefits.

Consider Margo Samson. She is a nurse who prides herself on her professionalism, compassion, and quality patient
care. She works side by side with Joan Finney, a nurse who is
widely perceived as unprofessional, rude, and inflexible. Margo
is painfully aware that Joan Finney's manager takes no action
to correct Joan's performance. This manager permits the standards and the reputation of the nursing service to be lowered,
which reflects on every nurse within the service. Margo is
demoralized; her pride in the organization fades.

And what about Lee, manager of the billing department. Lee has grown accustomed to mistakes in patients'
bills. The culprit is the computer, which spits out errors time
and again. Lee has come to tolerate billing errors and has
even staffed the department to handle the endless phone calls
from confused and angry customers inquiring about these
errors. Customers are dissatisfied, yet the billing errors have
become an accepted fact of life.

Tolerance of low standards means tolerance of mediocrity. Managers need to raise their standards in feasible, incremental steps.

Perhaps some managers are tolerant because they do
not have a vision of excellence. Others can envision excellence
but they do not want to confront employees who fall short for
fear of triggering rejection, insubordination, or job flight.
And perhaps they believe they can "get by" with less than
greatness because they always have. They rationalize that
because health care employees are such good people, they
must already be doing their best; pressing them to do better
will only make matters worse. Some managers are self-con-
scious about their own performance and feel unjustified in
expecting, from employees, performance that exceeds their
own. Many argue vociferously that excellence is not possible
in today's hectic and constraining environment. They claim

that it is hard enough to maintain the status quo, let alone raise standards!

Less tolerant managers on the other hand, those who insist on high standards and inch toward them, believe that if they do not monitor performance and press for improvements, backsliding is inevitable. They also have faith that their employees can stretch and improve. They know that tolerance of mediocrity will inevitably force the most talented and dedicated staff to leave for another employer who offers them a chance to feel proud. Employees with high standards lose heart when they see tears in the linen, litter on the floor, regular equipment breakdowns, and unnecessary expenditures because of neglect.

Managers with high standards communicate an ambitious vision, practice what they preach, appreciate others for excellence, and invest time and attention in building staff strengths.

Consider the issue of standards in three scenarios.

Case 1: James is a supervisor in your department. He has excellent technical skills, but displays poor interpersonal skills with patients and staff, consistently acting curt and abrupt. James is far short of a role model of excellence; however, he is never late, is never sick, and maintains a "this job is my life" attitude. When you confronted James in a low-key fashion, he was quick to blame co-workers for his abruptness, claiming that they made him irritable by failing to support him. A tolerant manager does not confront James for fear of alienating him or making him so angry that he leaves. Instead, the tolerant manager prefers to smooth the ruffled feathers created by James and justifies his inaction by adopting James's behavior of "blaming" others for his inappropriate behavior.

Managers committed to high standards handle this situation very differently. They do not tolerate James's behavior, because of the double message it sends to other employees and because it lowers the standards for the entire department. They confront James directly, citing specific examples and instances when James acted curt and abrupt. They are intent on helping James understand the importance of excellent performance and the consequences of continuing to act in an unacceptable manner. These managers may outline a "get well" plan with James and monitor his performance regularly.

Case 2: Nurses in your organization are under a great deal of pressure. Resources have been cut. Although positions remain unfilled, your staff must continue to care for the same number of patients. For your staff, these circumstances make lower quality standards for charting a foregone conclusion. When confronted about the incompleteness and errors in their charting, they complain about staffing, make excuses, and exclaim, "What do you expect?" This situation is not unusual in today's problem-fraught, lean environment. In response, tolerant managers feel forced to lower standards or just "get by." They accept the employees' excuses and feel helpless. Managers committed to excellence, however, respond differently. Some actively rethink charting to streamline it or help professionals chart more quickly without sacrificing quality (for example, dictaphones, more clerical support, predesigned checklists). Others insist that accurate, complete, and timely charting is an unequivocal priority and accept no excuses. In either case, these managers do not sit still. They hold to their standards tenaciously and tell employees point blank that stress is no excuse for slippage in chart quality.

Case 3: You are a vice-president. You have been in your job only six months. In that time, you have learned that Harriet, a department director who reports to you, is a thorn in your division's image. She is a long-term employee who has, over the years, developed a loyal following of co-workers and subordinates. You have been told by caring colleagues that any action to coach Harriet, change her job, or remove her from it will lead to an employee uprising. Yet, the pressure is on you, from your boss and Harriet's peers, to do something because she continues to tarnish your division's image. This is a sticky situation for any new manager, especially one who has entered with an inclination toward tolerance. Not wanting to create a scene, the tolerant manager ignores the situation and tells his boss that he has a "long-term" plan for dealing with Harriet "delicately." A new manager who wants to raise standards responds very differently. She lets staff know that she's planning to clarify her expectations for all department directors reporting to her. She meets with them to find out their perceptions of their own jobs and their expectations. She also takes time to learn the scuttlebutt on customers' perceptions of service and staff concerns about department management.

After building relationships with staff and learning the setup in the department, the vice-president calls a staff meeting. Now that she has heard each person's input and has had time to formulate her own expectations, she will meet with each person individually to clarify her expectations. She is alerting staff to the fact that she is the new vice-president and her expectations may be different from those that prevailed in the past. She sets up appointments and holds these meetings. When she meets with Harriet, she spells out in no uncertain terms what is expected. She does not talk about problem performance; she merely clarifies her own expectations and gives Harriet the chance to follow through. This vice-president knows that employees deserve to know what is expected of them before being dealt with as a problem employee. And this vice-president makes it very clear that she expects a lot. If time passes, and Harriet fails to meet the expectations, the vice-president will confront her and do everything necessary to bring performance up to standard or, if that proves impossible, to terminate Harriet.

What Is So Difficult About Raising Standards?

If high standards inspire pride, why do managers fail to raise the standards steadily? In our discussions, managers cite nine compelling reasons:

1. *Hopelessness:* You don't dare challenge the status quo around here when it comes to standards. If I tried to raise standards in my area, the myth of Sisyphus would take over. I would keep pushing the boulder up the mountain, and if I stopped for even a minute,

the boulder would roll back down. That's too
exhausting, so why try?

2. *Self-doubt:* I'll tell you the truth. I don't know
   if I have the skills or the guts to insist on
   higher standards.

3. *Empathy for employees:* My employees are
   under pressure. I don't feel right increasing
   my demands on them.

4. *Intimidation and fear of employee retaliation:*
   If I confront the problem people, I'll have to
   deal with their anger. I can hear it now—
   they'll feel unappreciated and abused. Then,
   I will have a worse morale problem on my
   hands.

5. *Ambivalence:* I'm just not convinced that raising standards in these times is the right thing
   to do. We don't have staff, time, or money.
   I'm not sure how much I can really expect.

6. *Work avoidance or fear of overwork:* If I push
   for more, it's going to mean more work for
   me. I'll have to look over people's shoulders,
   check their work, and work with them if I
   don't like what I see. That's work and I'm
   already working too hard.

7. *Fear about the ceiling on employee potential:*
   My staff are doing all they can now. I'd have
   to get different people if I wanted better performance. The thought of that gives me a
   migraine.

8. *Fear of being the outcast:* The standards aren't
   that high here. If I raised them for my
   people, I'd be out on a limb. I'd probably get
   razzed by other managers for brownnosing.

9. *Fear of dire negative consequences:* If I raise
   the standards, I could lose my job. It's just
   not politic around here to push the standards. The administrators won't support
   it.

Obviously, there are compelling reasons to leave the standards alone. You can leave at the end of the day feeling satisfied because you have accomplished your goals. You do not have to endure the discomfort, the unsettled feeling that accompanies the unfulfillable quest for constant improvement. You do not suffer the anxiety of confronting substandard performance or monitoring or coaching employees. And you can avoid the guilt derived from asking more of employees in these tough times.

When you leave the standards alone, the damage to staff motivation, productivity, work quality, and self-esteem and the effect on your organization's image and the outcomes for patients are even more compelling. We cannot afford anything less than continuously rising standards. Standards must move upward. If you are not trying to raise standards, they are probably slipping.

Mediocrity in today's marketplace means a declining market share as organizations increasingly compete on quality and service. Higher standards are an essential element in the formula for competitive success. Although the maintenance of high standards takes hard work, commitment, and energy, the payoffs are enormous for the organization and, in time, for you the manager. Lower standards mean lower performance; and that means more complaints from customers, more problems to solve, more fires to fight, in short, more, not less, work for you.

When you press for high standards, you retain your most talented people. They thrive on being part of a winning team. When you raise standards, you see improved performance, because most people have vast untapped potential. Many people grow and stretch in an atmosphere of higher expectations. This does not mean you should be unsympathetic or unfeeling. You can demand higher levels of performance and still empathize with employees. Managers who maintain high standards are respected by staff and superiors and are perceived as strong, not weak. You and your staff will be recognized and appreciated for your contributions.

What Strategies Can Be Used to Raise Standards?

To raise standards in your realm of influence, three strategies are essential: (1) resolve your mixed feelings about standards, (2) envision and talk excellence, (3) involve your staff in raising standards.

Strategy 1: Resolve your mixed feelings about standards. One recurrent reason for tolerance of mediocrity is mixed feelings on the part of the manager. Many managers are ambivalent about standards. On some days, they want employees to function better. On other days, they feel unjustified in expecting improved performance because people are too busy, stressed, or burnt-out.

Managers who have such mixed feelings cannot help but communicate them. As a result, employees know that higher levels of performance are not required. When the manager presses them to improve performance, they make the excuses that they know trigger the manager's mixed feelings.

Therefore, the standards remain fixed at a moderate level. Employees who perform at peak resent the fact that other employees are permitted to operate less effectively and, eventually, wonder why they should work so hard.

To resolve your mixed feelings, examine the performance that triggers them and make the tough decision to demand better performance. To raise standards, then, you need to render unacceptable some of the performance you have tolerated. You must narrow the gray area. Consider the continuum below.

Performance Continuum.

Unacceptable Performance	Gray Area	Acceptable Performance
←————————————————————————————————→		
50 percent error rate	10 percent error rate	1 percent error rate
Three-hour waits	Two-hour waits	Twenty-minute or shorter waits

Stealing, drinking on the job	Not smiling at patients	Listening with empathy, introducing self
Overspending by 50 percent	Overspending by 25 percent	Overspending by 5 percent
Insulting a patient	Interrupting, sounding rushed	Apologizing, offering assistance

In the left column is performance that is clearly unacceptable, and the right column, is clearly acceptable performance. The middle column—the gray area—is performance that the manager accepts some of the time and confronts some of the time—performance that triggers ambivalent feelings in the manager.

Not surprisingly, many aspects of performance are in the gray area. Some managers fail to confront employees for fear that the employee will retaliate with worse performance. Some managers question their right to expect so much. Others fear that any disciplinary action they take may be overturned, leaving the manager in an embarrassing position. Still others simply do not like to or do not have the skills to confront staff. Their self-image as humane and understanding makes confrontation very difficult or they cannot endure the stress associated with confrontation.

To raise standards, you need to make clear decisions about performance in the gray area and decide whether it is acceptable. You need to move mediocre performance from the gray area to the unacceptable realm and convey to staff your new and higher expectations.

To make these decisions, use the worksheet in Exhibit 2. Under Gray Area, list the types of performance currently under Gray about which you have mixed feelings. Then, consider each type long and hard, and decide whether it is acceptable. Eliminate the gray area.

Afterward, communicate your thoughts to staff. Explain that although they are doing a very good job, you believe they are capable of doing even better, and that customers deserve the very best. Emphasize that people have done

Exhibit 2. Decision Worksheet.

Unacceptable Performance	Gray Area	Acceptable Performance

nothing wrong—previous performance has been considered acceptable, but it will not be acceptable any longer. Reiterate why you feel it is important to raise standards and clarify your new expectations. Tell them you feel strongly that they deserve to hear from you a clear statement of what you expect. Present the new expectations. Invite reactions and discussion. Express confidence in your staff; tell them that now that they know what you expect, you know they will make every effort to achieve it. End by letting people know what you will do to support their efforts to meet the new expectations, for example, training, mentoring, coaching, feedback.

Consider two examples. First, imagine that patients are angered by the long waits in radiology. Typically, inpatients wait more than two hours as outpatients come and go. Rationalizations abound: inpatients have time on their hands and can afford to wait, ancillary scheduling for inpatients is complex, and so on. What is obvious is that patients miss meals when they wait a long time; they miss seeing their visitors; and they feel restless, anxious, and impatient. To heighten patient satisfaction, we should move tolerance of two-hour waits from the gray area into the area of unacceptability. Once the manager considers it unacceptable, he is likely to trigger substantive problem solving to improve scheduling or decrease waiting time for inpatients. Gray area performance is paralyzing; raised standards spark improvements.

Consider another example. Let us say your hospital is engaged in a service improvement strategy. Currently, your receptionist Mickey answers the phone in a friendly, helpful manner: "Hiya, what can I do for ya t'day?" Now that you have become aware of the behaviors that constitute excellent customer relations, you want her to sound more professional, for example, "Good morning, personnel, this is Mickey Robbins. How may I help you?"

You offer Mickey feedback during performance counseling and she responds: "Wait a minute. It says on my job description to be friendly and helpful and that's what I am." She is right. You realize that you need to communicate the change in your expectations. You rethink Mickey's job and lay out in great detail the service aspects. You add the following performance expectations to the position of receptionist to move Mickey toward "excellence":

• Greet customers with "Hello, personnel department. This is Mickey. How may I help you?" Smile and use a friendly tone.
• When a customer approaches you, tend to the customer immediately or let the customer know within fifteen seconds that you will be glad to help as soon as possible.
• Give clear directions and information, being careful not to use technical language or hospital jargon.
• If you do not know the answer to a customer's question, say that you will find the information and get back to him or her. Let the customer know how long it will take you to find out.

Then, sit down with Mickey to discuss the new expectations. Mickey needs you to affirm her previous efforts and at the same time express your seriousness about the new expectations. You can use the following approach for Mickey and your other employees:

1. Schedule a meeting with the employee. This meeting is similar to a performance appraisal meeting, so the same guidelines apply: privacy, adequate time for discussion, and so on.

2. Prior to the meeting, give the employee the new performance expectations so he or she can be prepared for the discussion.
3. Begin the discussion by giving the employee positive feedback on job performance. Even with "marginal" employees, you usually have observed some positive behavior: "John, I've noticed how hard you've been trying to move more quickly through your tasks." "Ann, I'm really pleased to hear you identifying yourself on the phone."
4. Review why you are raising and clarifying performance expectations.
5. Introduce and discuss the new performance expectations. Ask the employee for her or his *reaction* to the written expectations: "Are there any that seem unrealistic or inappropriate?" Help the employee anticipate the difficulties that may arise in fulfilling the expectations. Encourage the employee to identify specific situations that might be problematic.
6. Help the employee think through ways to handle these tough situations, so she or he will be able to fulfill your expectations, for example, how to remember to greet visitors with a pleasant tone and a smile even though three phone lines are ringing; how to calm an angry customer even though you already have a headache. For some employees, more than one meeting may be necessary. Remember that the purpose of this meeting is to help the employee move from "good" to "excellent" and some employees may need coaching.
7. Tell the employee to think about the expectations over the next few days and that you are available to help.
8. Confirm the discussion in writing.

A similar process works in situations where you want to clarify a new, higher standard for a formerly gray behavior. The following model developed by the Albert Einstein Healthcare Foundation outlines some effective steps:

Model for Communicating New Expectations

Step 1   Describe the past behavior that was formerly acceptable, in performance terms.

Step 2   Describe effects or consequences of the behavior.

Step 3   Express empathy.

Step 4   Make an "I expect" statement.

Describe the behavior in performance terms:

I want to talk with you about the incident this morning with Dr. Blakely. I was in my office and I could not help but overhear the words exchanged as well as observe the interaction. It was evident he was waiting to talk to you about his incomplete charts, and you failed to acknowledge his presence by continuing to talk on the phone, on what sounded like a personal phone call. Once you hung up, you did not look up, and in a flat monotone voice you said, "What do you need?" You did not address him by name, nor did your tone or actions demonstrate a willingness to help him.

Describe the effects or consequences of the behavior:

This lack of attention and indifferent treatment angered Dr. Blakely and immediately created a conflict that ended in his complaint to me. You know how hard we all work to get the doctors to properly complete their charts. Your behavior this morning is the very behavior that further antagonizes the doctors and makes it hard for us to obtain their cooperation.

Express empathy:

I recognize that not all doctors are easy to work with and that Dr. Blakely can be difficult. However . . .

Make an "I expect" statement:

Next time Dr. Blakely, or any physician, approaches your desk, I expect you to put aside whatever you are doing, including personal phone calls. I expect you to look up, smile, make eye contact, address the person by name, and ask what you can do in a positive, upbeat voice. In addition, I expect you to respond quickly to physicians' requests.

Use the following model the next time you become upset with an employee's behavior, a behavior that you know you have tolerated many times in the past.

1. Describe the specific situation and the employee's problem behavior.
2. Describe the consequences (for the customer, for the department, for the organization).
3. Offer empathy.
4. Clarify your expectations. What do you want from now on?

After clarifying new job-specific expectations, you need to document these in writing for yourself, the employee, and your human resources department, so that the employee cannot justifiably claim to have been unaware. Although documentation is time consuming and causes many managers anguish, it is a necessity if you want to hold people accountable to high standards and prevent your tough personnel decisions from being overturned later.

You can use this format to document the raising of standards:

1. Describe purpose of the memo: Summarize the new expec-

tations you communicated during your recent discussion with the employee.

2. Summarize background (prior discussions with the employee, incidents or problems leading up to your meeting).
3. Summarize the problem areas, including examples, their impact, and the employee's perception of those same incidents.
4. Restate your new and clearer expectations.
5. Summarize agreements reached (what the employee will do, what you and others will do to help, changes in work methods, the monitoring and feedback the employee can expect).
6. Share your optimism and confidence in the employee; state that this memo reflects your understanding of the recent discussion and invite the employee to respond if she or he was left with a different understanding.
7. Have the employee sign a copy to acknowledge receipt of the memo.

This strategy is grounded in reality: if you want the future to be different from the past in terms of standards, you have to differentiate past practices and outcomes that you tolerated from those you expect in the future. The past is over. Let us look ahead at the behavior needed *from now on.*

Of course, the same thinking applies to safety, health, and clinical quality standards.

Strategy 2: Envision and talk excellence. The second strategy that helps you to raise standards involves your own vision of excellence and communication of that vision with fervor and conviction to your staff.

Imagine two Eskimos sitting on chairs and fishing through holes in the ice. The Eskimo on the right drops his line through a typical small, disklike opening. The Eskimo on the left drops her line in the water too, and waits calmly for a nibble. This hole, however, is shaped like a crater; the opening extends to the horizon in the shape of a whale.

That is vision! The Eskimo on the left is ready. Her

fishing companion probably thinks she is eccentric and might even be critical: "How greedy can you get!" But, he cannot help but admit that his buddy is thinking big! From the very start of the project, this person has been a visionary.

And the vision is contagious. It is hard to sit very long beside a person with vision without enlarging your own vision.

You need to develop and articulate to your staff a clear mental picture of performance at the level you desire, a level higher than you currently tolerate. In short, the vision must inspire staff to work toward excellence. You cannot raise standards in your department unless you have a personal vision.

When we ask managers to role-play "excellence," most enact "fairly good" but not excellent behavior. And when asked to describe ways they would like their people to behave, managers usually depict nothing more ambitious or inspiring than "inoffensiveness." For instance, "I wish my staff wouldn't snap at patients," or "I wish we could get waiting time to under an hour." These images are not images of excellence. Inoffensiveness should not be acceptable. If you tolerate or are satisfied with inoffensiveness, you cannot challenge, excite, educate, or help your people stretch from "good" to "excellent." To elicit better performance, you need to help staff identify and seize opportunities and to incorporate new, improved behaviors into their everyday routine.

The vision of excellence starts with you. You formulate it in your mind, test its power to inspire on friends, and then communicate it to your employees and colleagues.

What is your vision? Take a sheet of paper and in five minutes describe how you want how your department/division to perform. Do not lift your pen from the paper; write as fast as you can, as much as you can, without attending to spelling or sentence structure. Push yourself to think big like the Eskimo woman.

After five minutes, stop writing. Read what you have written and ask yourself, "Am I inspired? Would this vision be worth fighting for?" If so, great! If not, try it again in a day or so. Put on some upbeat music, and push yourself again and again, until you have that vision of excellence.

Convene a meeting and ask your staff to perform the same exercise. Ask them to read their visions. Afterward, list the common themes. Examine the list with the group and ask people to identify those aspects of their visions that are within their immediate control. Form action plans to make the visions real. You will move one step closer to your vision. At the end of the meeting, articulate your own vision of excellence.

Visions or mental pictures of excellence are partly self-fulfilling. If you can picture higher performance, your staff will be much more likely to perform at a higher level. If you cannot communicate your vision to staff, how can you expect them to stretch beyond their current performance levels?

Strategy 3: Involve your staff in raising standards. The more you involve your staff in raising standards, the greater is their stake in upholding those standards. Staff meetings provide a natural forum in which to discuss and raise standards.

The "from good to great" meeting format is one way in which you can engage staff in raising standards, especially with respect to service.

"From good to great" meetings take as little as twenty minutes and have three important purposes: (1) to help your staff recognize the difference between "good" and "great" service-related performance; (2) to inspire staff toward greatness by helping them to identify and seize opportunities to satisfy customers; and (3) to provide much-needed practice in achieving excellence in everyday interactions with customers. The format for the "from good to great" meeting follows:

1. Explain the reasons for moving from "good" to "great" (heightened customer satisfaction, a positive grapevine about service quality, staff pride, and so on).
2. Divide staff into small groups of three or four.
3. Give each group a card that briefly describes a common interaction between your staff and customers. Proceed from the simple to the complex. Start with "greeting a patient warmly" and move to "entering an AIDS patient's

room to find that the patient is asleep and his mother is sitting there crying." Brainstorm situations in advance with staff. One list can last for many meetings. Note these situations:

- Staff coming across a lost person in the hall
- Service person changing a light bulb in a patient's room
- Purchasing staff contacting department head to reject a requisition that was improperly submitted
- Technician explaining a long wait to a patient in X ray
- Employee delivering a food tray to a patient with arthritic hands
- An employee saying "no" to a patient because the patient's request violates the hospital's safety policy
- Employee receiving a phone call meant for another department
- Nurse walking in on a visitor who is upset

4. Clarify the task. Each small group should stage two one-minute skits. The first skit should portray a poor response to the assigned situation; the second skit should portray an excellent response to the same situation. The idea is to define the two extremes on the behavior continuum for the particular situation.
5. After a five-minute planning period, have the groups perform their skits. On the wall post two questions they should consider after viewing the skits: What behaviors were great? What *other* behaviors might have made the employee's performance even better?
6. Reconvene the entire group and ask how easy or hard it was to be great. Emphasize that it is not hard to be good, and most people are, but, to be *great*, a person must consciously work to identify opportunities, seize those opportunities, and then integrate the newly acquired behavior into the everyday routine.

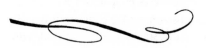

4

From Directing
to Empowering Your Staff

1. Do you expect your employees to adhere to policies and procedures in all circumstances? YES NO
2. Do you believe managers and supervisors are the only people who should make exceptions to rules? YES NO
3. Do you think you should do all you can to shelter your employees from unpleasant situations? YES NO
4. Do you feel more gratified when you solve problems for your employees than when they solve them without your help? YES NO
5. Do you feel insecure at the thought that your people can function very well without you? YES NO
6. Do you feel proud of your employees when they bend the rules creatively to satisfy a customer's needs? YES NO
7. Do you pour energy into helping your staff make increasingly important and responsible decisions? YES NO

8. Do you see your role as enabling your
    employees to serve their customers?   YES   NO
9. Do you help your employees learn to make
    judgments on the front lines without gain-
    ing your permission?   YES   NO
10. If an employee has a problem, are you more
    likely to ask for his or her ideas about a
    solution than you are to intervene with
    yours?   YES   NO

Add the number of "no" responses to the first five questions to the number of "yes" responses to the last five questions. The higher your score, the more you see your role as
that of empowering rather than directing employees.

In the past, when status quo management was the
norm, it made sense for managers to direct employees to per-
petuate practices. With the customer at the bottom of the
power pyramid, there was little need to adapt rules, regulations, policies, and procedures. If there were problems with
patients, physicians, or colleagues, the manager intervened to
solve the problem. Employees were not expected to step in
and solve problems or bend rules to satisfy customers while
still protecting the needs of the organization.

Those days are gone. With the increasing emphasis on
meeting customer needs and outcompeting your rivals, frontline employees are pressured from all directions to perform
differently—to go the extra mile, to bend rules in certain circumstances, to make reparations in the face of complaints, to
do whatever it takes to achieve customer satisfaction.

It sounds simple, but it is not easy, because employees
are accustomed to directive managers who do not teach
employees to make judgments on their own. Employees need
the *latitude* to make decisions on behalf of their customers,
and, in most health care organizations, rules, regulations,
safety precautions, and especially management practices have
not provided this latitude.

Extensive red tape interferes with the empowerment of
employees. If a patient does not receive a meal or is brought

the wrong food, the first employee who learns of this should be able to remedy the situation. A system must be in place to support that employee. In most service-oriented businesses, employees have such power, but not in health care.

If we want employees to take the initiative to satisfy our customers, then they must have the power and freedom to do so. And they must be allowed to make mistakes. When employees are unable to act because they have to ask their bosses, delays, indecisiveness, and missed opportunities rule. Managers must provide their staff with the proper training and then allow them to act. If they should err, the manager's response should not be a reproach. The manager should thank the employee for taking action, back him up, and discuss with him how the problem could have been handled more effectively.

To empower employees, management style must change from directing and controlling to *empowering*.

Directive managers tell their employees what to do in great detail. They see their main job as keeping employees in line and, in the face of problems, supporting their employees by intervening and solving these problems. They need to approve all deviations from standard practice and ensure that employees ask permission before taking initiatives that involve other people or resources.

Empowering managers encourage employees to exercise their own judgment even if it means special effort. They urge employees to take the initiative to make their own jobs more effective, to solve problems, and to enhance service at their own level without permission or advice from their manager. The empowering manager supports employees by coaching them on their options and negotiating with them the latitude within which they can act. Empowering managers remove the obstacles that prevent employees from performing their jobs effectively and without frustration. Knowing that people will learn from experience, the empowering manager offers lavish praise for even imperfect attempts to take initiative.

In summary, the shift from director to empowerer is a radical shift in mindset on the part of the manager from

"What can you do for me?" to "What can I do to enable you
to do your job effectively?"

*Case 1: You have just been notified of the due date for
submitting capital budget needs and the required proposals.
You are aware that many different people in your department
have equipment needs.* The directive manager asks employees
to suggest equipment needs and explain why this equipment
is needed. Then, this manager develops the required proposals and determines the priorities.

The empowering manager also invites employees to
identify these needs. But this manager goes further and
involves employees in the proposal and prioritization, believing that involvement in this process will make them better
able to grasp departmental finances, understand competing
needs, and develop the ability to evaluate difficult trade-offs.

*Case 2: One of your long-term employees tends to become
dysfunctional and hostile when under pressure. He has been
known to snap at physicians and has caused numerous complaints.* The directive manager tells this employee that such
behavior is unacceptable and perhaps disciplines the employee. Or, she might alter the employee's job by preventing
him from interacting extensively with physicians.

An empowering manager takes a more positive approach. She helps the employee and other staff to generate
alternative ways to handle difficult interactions and difficult
customers. This manager counsels the employee about how
to interact with physicians more effectively and perhaps
invests in the employee's development by sending him to a
workshop on dealing with difficult people. The manager
expects a change in behavior and encourages the employee to
develop the skills needed to make the change.

*Case 3: A patient complained vociferously about a
recent meal. Upon hearing the complaint, an employee apolo-
gized for the poor-quality food on behalf of the organization
and insisted on obtaining another meal for the patient. The
dietary department was able to provide this meal, but was
inconvenienced by the request.* The directive manager expresses his annoyance with the employee that she promised

the patient a replacement meal without first consulting him. The empowering manager thanks the employee for resolving the patient's complaint. He appreciates that she went out of her way to satisfy the patient. Because this action did inconvenience other staff, the manager discusses with the employee alternative responses to such a complaint, if any exist. The point here is to reinforce employee initiative, coach the employee to make better judgments, and intervene with other people and departments to make sure that they back up the frontline employee's promises to patients even if they are inconvenienced. The empowering manager realizes that this employee is precious because of her commitment to satisfying the patient.

Case 4: One of your employees gets into a fight with a co-worker, causing quite a scene in the work area. The directive manager counsels both people independently, making it clear that their behavior was inappropriate. The empowering manager is more likely to bring the two employees together to work out their differences, before he intervenes. If the employees cannot, the manager insists on mediating a dialogue between the two, pushing them to agree with one another before he dictates how the conflict must be resolved.

There are many good reasons for encouraging employees to be proactive and independent. You cannot be everywhere at the same time and the organization needs your people to focus on the customer. Your people need to know how far they can go to please customers. And they need to know that you will back them up even when they make mistakes.

Obstacles

Making the shift from directive to empowering manager is not easy because the directive style has many advantages. As you are ultimately responsible for what happens in your area, you might feel in much more control if you are directive. You may fear that if you give up some of your control and enable employees to make more independent decisions, you will no longer know what is going on and be "out of control." This can be extremely uncomfortable for managers with superiors who want to be updated at a moment's notice. For many managers, responding "I don't know" is paramount to admitting "I can't control my people or my department." Many managers feel successful *only* when they know every detail.

You may feel "vital" to your staff and to the organization when your employees come to you for solutions and advice. You also might enjoy the attention. When employees need you to solve their problems, they worry about "getting in good" with you, so they can rely on you to help them when they need help.

Also, empowering requires considerable time, especially in the short term. If you loosen control and empower your staff, you will have to endure their mistakes, because no one is perfect and you are ultimately responsible. When you have to intervene, and you will, you may feel that you should have handled the problem by yourself from the beginning. You also need to devote time to staff development so that your staff are able to handle situations appropriately and creatively.

Benefits

Are there compensatory benefits? Absolutely. Without a doubt, your employees will be able to handle more and you will, in time, gain greater control over your own time. Staff will feel more energized and less mechanical. They will feel better about their performance and their value to the organization. They will use each other as resources because they do not have to use you. Finally, you will not feel trapped. You can take that sick day, attend that conference, and work on that special project.

Today, you cannot afford to have your people utterly dependent on you. Such dependence impedes their personal growth and creativity. Bottlenecks at your desk are inefficient and wasteful, delaying the services delivered by your staff. Only through empowerment do you build ownership and commitment. And only through empowerment do you increase productivity.

Strategies

Empowering managers involve employees in substantive issues. They enlist their support in formulating solutions. They enable them to do the job by providing them with the tools, resources, and skills needed to do the job right. Further, they communicate their value and respect for staff efforts by offering encouragement and recognition.

Four simple, yet far-reaching strategies translate these characteristics into action: (1) Solicit input from your employees by providing regular "input opportunities." (2) Help employees exercise sound judgment in choice situations. (3) Replace obstacles with backup systems. (4) Coach; do not supply answers.

Strategy 1: Solicit input from your employees by providing regular "input opportunities." The first step in empowering employees is to invite their input on a regular basis. Routinely encourage employees to think for the department and for the organization, to help you consider opportunities and problems that extend beyond their specific jobs. By inviting their input, you not only benefit from their perspectives; you also provide employees with invaluable experience.

The input can pertain to any topic about which a decision must be made, for example:

- How can we improve our work environment?
- What can we do to improve relationships with department X?
- How can our organization differentiate itself from the hospital up the street?
- How can we improve our recognition practices?
- Which procedures of this department annoy our customers? What can we do to change?

Many managers hesitate to invite employee input because they fear hearing what they do not want to hear and being unable to respond to the issues raised in a manner that maintains employee trust and builds their own credibility.

You can prevent these fears from becoming realities by design, by creating opportunities for employees to make constructive contributions, and by handling their ideas and concerns credibly.

Exhibit 3 illustrates an invitation to an input meeting that worked very well, because it was designed carefully and focused on a "real" need. Employees knew what was expected of them and prepared to be full participants in the meeting.

Exhibit 3. Invitation to an Input Meeting.

To: All staff
Re: September 15th Staff Meeting

As you know, we are holding a special staff meeting Tuesday afternoon, September 15th, from 1:00 to 3:30 P.M. The purpose is to examine our scheduling procedures for outpatients. We currently allow fifteen minutes per patient visit. Many people say that this might not be the best approach for both patients and staff. This meeting will be a bit longer than usual so that we have enough time to discuss this important subject.

So that we can use the meeting time effectively, please do the following beforehand:

• List the patients to whom you are assigned between now and the meeting and their specific conditions.
• Look over your schedule charts and determine which patients/conditions need more or less than the fifteen minutes allotted.
• [For receptionists] Between now and the meeting, record the number of patients seen on time and keep track of how long others have to wait, so we can see our problem in greater detail. Bring the results with you to the meeting. I will be glad to help you work out a format for tracking.

With this information, I know we will be able to define the problem clearly and discuss ways to improve our system. If we can improve scheduling, I am convinced that patients will be happier and staff will be less frustrated.

See you then! I am looking forward to it.

At the meeting, the manager began with this introduction:

Your questions tell me that all of you received my memo last week. Some of you expressed nervousness about making changes in scheduling because so many items will be affected. That is true. Frankly, I am nervous about it too. But the fact is that our patients have not been well served by the current system, as you can tell from the many complaints.

We will not make a change unless we research it carefully and develop what we believe is a solid, workable plan in which we have confidence. We will not change for the sake of change.

Today, I ask you to share the information you brought to the meeting and your views of our current system. For the first half hour, each person will speak for a few minutes, summarizing his or her findings. We will then have twenty minutes for open discussion. In the half hour that remains, we will determine which alternatives might better serve our patients and us. We will not make any decisions today. We will generate ideas into which a small group of us will look further after the meeting. Then, in two weeks, I will report back to you our recommendations for further discussion.

I need your help and support in this effort. I hope that you will be candid and involved in today's meeting.

One department head complained, "I sent out a memo letting my staff know that I wanted to hold a meeting to discuss new ways to follow up on our patients. I wanted staff input before I made any decisions that would affect them. I outlined the situation—what was not working from the patient's perspective—and asked for reactions. No one spoke up. There was not one idea in the group; of course, after the meeting, they had a great deal to say, mostly criticisms. What did I do wrong?"

Often, employees are reluctant to share ideas and suggestions in a large group. They are afraid to say something foolish or controversial. It is helpful to divide them into smaller groups (of two, three, or four), because small groups are safe. Give the group focused questions and specify the amount of time they have for discussion. Ask each group to name a person to record comments and report back to the whole group at the end. Small groups encourage more people to speak up. They also avoid putting people on the spot.

Of course, when the small groups report their results to the whole group, they will take their cues from you as facilitator. Your willingness to listen and accept their ideas will determine how open they are.

Convene an input meeting monthly. This tells your employees that their concerns are important enough to warrant regular time and attention.

Strategy 2: Help employees exercise sound judgment in choice situations. Many managers fail to empower their employees because they do not trust their employees to act wisely. You can minimize the risk of unwise judgments on the part of your employees by deliberately helping them examine alternative, appropriate responses to a variety of situations.

At staff meetings, divide the group into small subgroups. Give each subgroup a case study for which it must generate appropriate responses. Afterward, the subgroups can share their approaches and get feedback. You then have an opportunity to add your comments. Here are ten practice situations you can use:

1. Ninety-year-old Mrs. Brown has serious heart trouble and has been admitted to the hospital several times in the past year. Her daughter has signed a do-not-resuscitate (DNR) form each time and you are aware that both the patient and her daughter have asked the doctors involved not to use extreme measures if Mrs. Brown experiences heart failure. Mrs. Brown has been admitted today and you notice that the DNR form has not been signed.

2. Your boss asks you to evaluate two vendors and to recommend the vendor you think the department should

use. After investigating both vendors, you realize that neither provides the service required.

3. You need an O-ring for an elderly patient. You have called the storeroom and they are back-ordered. You have called other floors and none is available. The patient really needs this item.

4. Mrs. Jones's daughter is upset with you because her mother's personal belongings have disappeared. Mrs. Jones is not your patient and her nurse is away on vacation.

5. You are a supervisor in environmental services. One day, because of absenteeism, you do not have enough staff to set up rooms for all the special functions scheduled.

6. You work in maintenance. You stopped in a room to replace a doorknob and the patient asks you to install a stronger light bulb in the lamp. You need a work order to change a light bulb.

7. You are a technician. Suddenly, the equipment breaks down. Many patients are waiting. You cannot find a supervisor.

8. Bob Smith has been admitted through the emergency room. His clothes were ripped and covered with blood when he arrived in the ambulance. They have been discarded.

9. Charlie Hertz has been at his father's bedside since he was brought into the hospital. Every time you suggest that Charlie take a break to get some food or coffee, he refuses. You know he has not eaten in at least six hours.

10. A patient has traveled a long distance for a test. Unfortunately, this patient is not scheduled until the next day.

After working on the practice situations, ask employees to share real situations that they have found difficult to handle. Ask them to write them down on a slip of paper. Place the slips of paper in a hat. Have individuals draw situations at random and role-play or discuss their proposed solutions.

The benefit of this approach is that employees solve their *own* problems. To handle situations well, employees require good judgment *and* the latitude to act. As you explore each situation, examine in detail the degree to which the employee can bend rules. Many employees have great ideas about how to handle situations, but they feel constrained by rules and the confines of their job descriptions. Reexamine the latitude you have given employees to use their judgment to satisfy customers. They will not act if you discourage their actions by placing obstacles at every turn.

Strategy 3: Replace obstacles with backup systems. When employees consider alternatives, they are quick to point to the obstacles that interfere with their ability to act. Sure, some employees might decide to send the indigent patient home in hospital scrubs (situation 8 in the preceding list of practice situations), or might extend their breaks and run to the hospital supply store to buy an O-ring for the elderly patient (situation 3 in the same list).

To empower your employees, you must identify the obstacles that prevent them from taking initiative and making decisions. You must enable them to act instead. Employees cite the following major impediments to their empowerment:

1. *Red tape:* I know what to do, but I can't do it on the spot because of all the hoops you have to go through to get anything done here.
2. *Punitiveness:* My boss is quick to berate me if I do something that he doesn't think was the best thing to do for that patient. I figure it's not worth the risk to stick my neck out by bending the rules even if I believe it's the best thing for the patient and for our organization.
3. *Unclear communication lines for follow-through:* Most of the time, I can think of what needs to be done to satisfy somebody's need, but I don't have the power to do it by myself. I might need to pull in another department or other people and I certainly do not have the authority to do that. If I asked someone in another department to do

something for a patient without going through my boss, that person would think I had really overstepped.

4. *Inadequate systems for following through on nonroutine requests:* I don't dare promise a patient anything special, because I couldn't get people to deliver on my promise. I wouldn't know who to call, where to go, or how to go about getting a special need met. And if I ask the people I think could help, they are annoyed because it's not their job.

5. *Management ambivalence about letting go of control:* My boss says to take initiative and make decisions at my level, but it's a laugh. He is threatened unless I go through him. I think he needs to feel that he's the power-house and that without his permission, nothing happens.

6. *No resources available to support initiatives:* I wanted to give the patient scrubs to wear home, so he wouldn't have to wear his torn, bloody clothes, but I know it costs the department money. So what do I do?

All of these obstacles reduce employee decisiveness, initiative, and action on behalf of customers. To empower employees, eliminate these impediments.

Cut the red tape. Determine legitimate ways in which employees can short-circuit cumbersome approval processes, or bend the rules, and act on the customer's behalf expeditiously. If a maintenance worker is stopped by a patient who asks for a higher-wattage light bulb, he should be able to fulfill that request immediately. The patient should not have to wait days while the employee submits a work order for approval by superiors. Perhaps, you might identify certain "quick action" tasks that employees can handle without approval or set an expenditure level below which employees can make decisions on their own.

Appreciate, do not punish, employees who take inappropriate actions. At Delta and SAS airlines, employees have substantial power to act on their own to satisfy customers. An employee who encounters a disgruntled passenger has considerable latitude to rectify the problem or make reparations (in some cases, even offer a free air ticket for future use). If the employee exercises this freedom at great cost to the company (for example, "I'm sorry, ma'am. Let me see to it that you receive four free tickets to Hawaii!"), the supervisor does not berate the employee; instead, she thanks the person for turning a disgruntled customer into a loyal customer. Then, she suggests alternative, less costly solutions. The employee is appreciated, not punished. You cannot encourage employees to think on their own and make decisions if you punish them for every decision you dislike. You need to encourage them to become stronger and make more appropriate judgments.

Clarify the appropriate communication lines for follow-through: If a patient asks a housekeeper for different food, who does that housekeeper call? The head nurse, the housekeeper's supervisor, the dietitian, the patient representative? In many organizations, employees do not act because they do not know whom to contact. This lack of knowledge makes follow-through very time consuming. Each employee should know those people he or she can use as resources in different situations. If employees must locate their supervisors and vie for their attention, then the employee is not empowered.

Design systems that employees can use to follow through on nonroutine requests. You need to think through and design processes that allow employees to act quickly.

Confront and resolve your ambivalence about letting go of control. Consider your own feelings about control. If you must retain control of every move an employee makes to feel worthy, then stop talking about empowerment. It frustrates employees when their managers talk empowerment but then fail to give them the freedom to act. If you have a problem with control but you want to overcome it, try admitting this to your employees. Ask them to bring up the control issue when they feel you are limiting their freedom to act.

Allocate funds or locate (for example, from the auxiliary, volunteers, development office) discretionary resources to encourage constructive employee initiative. Some resources should be available so that employees can let an occasional patient go home in scrubs, buy extra O-rings, provide a celebration pizza, or mail a caring follow-up card after patient discharge. Consider a slush fund (with a *simple* approval process) that employees can tap when they want to do something for a customer. The resource pool does not have to be enormous.

Your employees will energetically formulate alternatives and act on them if they believe you will back them up with systems, effort, and resources.

Strategy 4: Coach; do not supply answers. To develop effective, independent decision makers, you must resist the temptation to think for employees. They must think for themselves. Help employees to think through alternatives, to develop criteria on which to base decisions, and to apply these criteria to actual situations; however, you must stop having all the answers and press employees to do the thinking.

Sara, a nurse in the emergency room, recognized the unusual level of fear expressed by a family over the status of their teenage son who had just been in a motorcycle accident. Sara felt strongly that the family would calm down if their doctor were there to reassure them. Because Sara believed that the doctor would not make the trip to the hospital simply to reassure the family, she exaggerated the status of the boy on the phone, forcing the physician to hurry to the hospital.

Anne, Sara's manager, did not berate her or tell her how to handle such situations in the future. Instead, she helped Sara rethink the situation and develop a more effective approach.

Anne: What were you trying to achieve by calling Dr. Parks?

Sara: I wanted him to speak with the family. I felt that the patient, the family, and all of us in the emergency room needed him there.

Anne: And did you get what you wanted?

Sara: He came. He spoke with the family. He put them at ease. Of course he snapped at me, but that's Dr. Parks.

Anne: How did you get him to come? What did you tell him?

Sara: I told him that we had a very sick child and a frightened family and we needed him. Why are you asking me?

Anne: Dr. Parks told me that you called him to come over and that he was glad you did, but he said that you sounded hysterical "as usual."

Sara: I wanted him here for the sake of the family. Does it matter how I got him here?

Anne: What do you think?

Sara: Not to the patient.

Anne: How about for you and your relationship with the physician? How about for us—the rest of us who need to have a good relationship with and respect from Dr. Parks. We need to have him work with us and trust us.

Sara: So what should I have done?

Anne: Think about it. Think about why you really needed him to come. Was it for the patient? For the family? For you?

Sara: Mostly for the family, but I led him to believe that the patient needed him.

Anne: And what effect did that have?

Sara: I guess he saw through me when he saw the patient and met the family. It was obvious who needed him the most. But I just didn't feel he would care or come if I told him the truth. Doctors don't care about the family as much as the patient.

Anne: I think you're prejudging this doctor.

Sara: I guess so, but there is a long history to support me.

Anne: I'd like you to try other approaches in the future, approaches that might be more effective in maintaining the physician's trust. Can you think of any other approaches?

Sara: I could have said, "Dr. Parks, a young teenager was just brought in with a fractured skull. Your resident is doing everything he can but the parents are very upset. I think they are making it harder on the boy and I know they are putting pressure on your resident. There is family history in this case that makes their behavior understandable, but I don't believe that we can help them. I think they need to hear from you that their son will survive and what you will be doing in the next forty-eight hours."

Anne: How does that sound to you?

Sara: Actually, that sounded pretty good. It would be nice not to have to play games with doctors so much.

Anne: I agree. I'm hoping you'll try that kind of approach in the future. You know, while I think this approach would be better for all concerned, I still want you to know that I appreciate your great concern for the family in this instance and realize that you were doing all you could to give them what you thought they needed. I am very grateful for your dedication to your patients and know how far you will go to help them. You are a role model for our team.

Sara: Thanks and I'll try a different tack next time.

Help your employees to generate alternative solutions to problems that arise in their jobs. How? The next time a problem arises that you think could have been handled better, use the following guide:

1. Thank the employee for handling the situation independently.

2. Ask the employee to replay the situation and evaluate the outcomes.
3. Ask the employee to identify preferable outcomes.
4. Encourage the employee to think of other ways such situations can be addressed to bring about those preferable outcomes. Press the employee to do the thinking. Offer suggestions but not too quickly.
5. Ask the employee to evaluate the strengths and possible negative consequences of each alternative. Add your own thoughts here, but not too quickly.
6. End by asking the employee to summarize what he or she thinks would be the best approach in future situations, based on this discussion.

Power is vastly different from control. To increase your power in the organization, you need to loosen the reins and give employees the freedom to act creatively to accomplish their tasks and satisfy customers. Employees with great potential will be energized and increase their contributions to the organization. You are responsible for the results achieved in your area. If you let go and enable your employees to act, your status will be enhanced by their accomplishments.

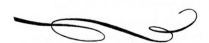

5

From Employee as Expendable Resource to Employee as Customer

1. Do you consider your employees as customers whose satisfaction is key to the success of your organization?   YES   NO
2. After observing you during a routine day, would others conclude that you take for granted your employees' dedication to their jobs?   YES   NO
3. Do you have a conscious, deliberate strategy in place to identify employee needs and work to satisfy them as your key customers?   YES   NO
4. Do you balk at employee demands because you think employees should be grateful for what they are already getting from work?   YES   NO
5. Do you think that employee involvement and participation are more a matter of necessity than a matter of style?   YES   NO
6. Do you resent the time it takes to nurture and support employees?   YES   NO
7. Do you devote more time and energy to retention of good staff than you devote to recruitment of new people?   YES   NO

8. Do you think money is the main factor that
    affects employee satisfaction and retention?   YES   NO

If you answered "yes" to any of the odd-numbered
questions and "no" to any of the even-numbered questions,
you perceive employees as scarce and valuable resources whose
satisfaction and well-being you need to cultivate deliberately
and conscientiously. This contrasts with the perception that
employees are essentially replaceable and even dispensable,
that you can find good people if the ones you have do not
meet standards or do not like the job.

As the service sector expands, service industries, especially hotels, airlines, restaurants, and, yes, health care organizations, are suffering worker shortages. Staffing shortages
are worse in health care because they extend across a wide
range of unskilled and professional-technical specialties.

Health care has been hit harder than other industries
for several reasons. Women, traditionally drawn to health
care, now find that other avenues are open to them. Salaries
in certain clinical and technical areas, such as nursing, physical and respiratory therapy, pharmacy, and radiology, have
not remained competitive, so people turn to other professions
to expand their earning potential and growth opportunities.
Also, health care workers leave because their formerly stable
workplaces are now chaotic, frustrating, and insecure. Fear
and paranoia related to AIDS and other contagious and life-
threatening diseases and increasingly discordant and stressful
relationships between physicians and nonphysicians, between
patients and staff, and among co-workers have accelerated job
flight. The status ascribed to health care workers has, in the
view of many, sharply declined as the media lambast health
care organizations for skyrocketing costs, ethical problems,
malpractice, and questionable quality of care.

Employees, especially those inclined toward the helping
professions, desire more than decent salaries and benefits.
They seek the support needed to make a substantial contribution. They want to feel a sense of accomplishment, of belonging, and of pride in the organization's standards and quality

care. Preoccupied by turmoil and rapid change, health care employers are hard put to give employees what they want and need to remain productive on the job and loyal to the organization. Too often, workers feel frustrated. Their once touted "ideal job" is not seen as ideal anymore. Not only do they feel frustrated, isolated, overworked, and undervalued, but they are spreading the word and dissuading others from entering the health care professions.

At a recent workshop for nursing supervisors, one manager remarked, while others nodded in assent, that "I'd do anything to talk my kids out of getting into health care. It just isn't worth it."

The implications for managers? It is difficult, sometimes desperately difficult, to attract and retain good people. And, because we are talking about health care, the consequences range from debilitating to hazardous. You cannot run a hospital without sufficient staff. You cannot be successful unless you have a dependable team. Devoting time and energy to hiring without providing the training, development, nurturing, and opportunity necessary to retain the good people you already have is like running the water with the drain open.

You need to think of employees as indispensable and irreplaceable and adjust your priorities and practices to cultivate their effectiveness and loyalty.

Different Managerial Types

Managers who recognize the difficulty of replacing employees and who value their employees' talent and dedication as their greatest asset spend their time and attention differently from managers who do not. They are attuned to employee needs and concerns. They train their people to do the job well, in line with high standards, and provide the tools needed to perform without frustration. They foster harmonious, supportive relationships among their staff, building teamwork and a sense of family that earns employee loyalty. They offer employees meaningful opportunities to participate in quality

improvement and work-life decisions to increase their gratifi-
cation by increasing their contribution to the group and the
organization. They allocate time and resources toward improving the environment for employees and enhancing their quality of work life. They are generous with appreciation and
acknowledgment. In short, they work hard to help employees
feel cared for and special.

Managers who view employees as replaceable or expend-
able feel and act quite differently. They take employees for
granted and do not devote time to nurturing. Many of these
managers think employees are too picky and demanding and
that "if you give them an inch, they'll take a mile." Some
believe that you cannot change people, motivate them, or
improve their performance—"they either have it or they
don't." As a consequence of these attitudes, management
practices deprive employees of the support, coaching, feedback, nurturing, appreciation, participation, and respect they
need to persevere in their increasingly stressful and difficult
jobs.

*Case 1: You notice that several people you supervise are
not working well together. They complain about one another's
performance, spread rumors, and avoid talking directly with
one another.* Managers who minimize the importance of invest-
ing in employees try to eliminate the offenders: "a couple of
rotten apples can spoil the barrel." Or they might deny the
impact of disharmony in their desire to avoid confrontation
of the problem or the people involved and hope that the problem will pass or the people will habituate to it.

Managers who perceive employees as valuable and irreplaceable respond differently. They confront the problem
together with their staff, help people to communicate directly
with one another and come to terms, and then develop a
follow-up plan to prevent such problems and sustain harmonious co-worker relationships.

*Case 2: Your employees are so different with respect to
their interests, values, and life-styles that it is excruciatingly
difficult to plan special events that satisfy everyone.* This common problem frustrates many managers. Managers who see

employees as replaceable either eliminate special events because "they're just too much trouble" or make expedient decisions to sponsor infrequent, low-effort events as symbolic tokens of togetherness, even if these events do little to build cohesion or communicate appreciation. Employee-focused managers go further and choose locations, foods, and activities that appeal to the majority. This frequently entails an enormous amount of work, but the payoff in employee investment and support is worth it.

Case 3: Through the grapevine you hear that department morale is down. You feel that you have done everything possible to listen to and support your employees and are extremely frustrated. Managers who treat employees as replaceable often resent the time and energy already spent on improving employee morale. They may pinpoint the small number of employees who instigated the problem and eliminate them. Or they may ignore the problem, rationalizing that it is par for the course in any workplace and probably not amenable to change. These managers are impatient with employees: "They're here to do a job; why can't they just do it without all this fuss?" Their impatience and anger spill over to employees and aggravate the morale problem.

Other managers recognize employees as customers whose satisfaction matters to the organization. These managers acknowledge the delicate *balance* between what the employee can do for the organization and what the organization can do for the employee. They express concern about morale problems and do their best to lift morale by meeting with staff, forming work-life task forces, bringing in an outsider to conduct team building or problem analysis, and more. They might, for instance, convene a meeting to "take the pulse" of the staff, holding an open, nondefensive stance and inviting the staff's perspectives and solutions. In other words, they devote time and energy to investigating and relieving the problem. They are not satisfied to let it be, because it erodes employee productivity, satisfaction, and longevity. They view time spent on bolstering morale as a prudent investment.

Strategies That Strengthen Employee Loyalty

You have probably heard of Frederick Herzberg's research on motivation. According to Herzberg (1987), two types of factors affect employee satisfaction: "hygiene factors" and "motivation factors." Hygiene factors must be present for employees to avoid feeling actively dissatisfied; however, motivation factors must be present for employees to feel actively motivated and satisfied with their work. Here are examples (Herzberg, 1987, p. 112):

Hygiene Factors	*Motivation Factors*
Company policy	Achievement
Supervision	Recognition
Work conditions	Work itself
Salary	Responsibility
Relationship with peers	Advancement

If you eliminate the hygiene factors that dissatisfy, people are no longer unhappy, but neither are they happy. If workers are to be happy, the motivation factors must be harnessed. This means that managers who want to satisfy employee needs and retain their loyalty must deliberately cultivate employee satisfaction.

As a result of focus groups we held with diverse groups of hospital employees, we have come to see the critical motivation factors as somewhat different for health care employees who are, on the whole, idealistic individuals who chose health care because of their people orientation and desire to help others. Employees identified the following as their burning needs:

Bonding and belonging: Feelings of connectedness and harmony must be fostered among staff. Help your staff to know one another on both a personal and a professional basis and work with them to build harmony, interdependence, and support.

Appreciation and recognition for a job well done: Employees value most the very simple pat on the back from their supervisors and co-workers. Managers must acknowledge employees often and genuinely.

Contribution: Employees want to do a good job and contribute to patient care.

Le Boeuf (1985, pp. 88–89) in *The Greatest Management Principle in the World* talks about the most important words in our language:

The five most important words are "You did a good job."
The four most important words are "What is your opinion?"
The three most important words are "Let's work together."
The two most important words are "Thank you."
The single most important word is "We."

We now provide five strategies you can use to address these employee needs and thereby translate your dedication to your employees into action: (1) Create a close, supportive team. (2) Cultivate smooth co-worker relationships. (3) Learn the language of appreciation and use it. (4) Spark a sense of contribution by sharing responsibility for your group's health. (5) Monitor employee satisfaction and use the results to hold yourself accountable.

Strategy 1: Create a close, supportive team. On-the-job cooperation and spirited teamwork are rooted in personal understanding and mutual support. You can use structured techniques and exercises, in staff meetings or at birthday parties or other special events, to promote such understanding and support within your own department or division. Such activities transform staff meetings from information-giving sessions that foster passivity to participatory experiences that invite active communication. They create memorable team-building experiences that help your staff feel appreciated. And they cultivate communication and cooperation among your employees.

Icebreakers/meeting openers are quick (ten to twenty minutes) methods for starting meetings that help your staff focus on one another as people. To open, say something such as "Before we focus on the business of today's meeting, I think it would be nice to take a few minutes to focus on how we're doing as people." Then, try one of these people-connecting warmups:

Taking the pulse: Write the following words on a flipchart or chalkboard: *soaring, sailing, swimming, sinking.* Ask group members to select one or more of these words to describe how they have been feeling lately on or off the job. They can use another word if none of these fits. Ask a volunteer to share his or her word and the reason for choosing it. Continue with the person to the left or right of the employee who just spoke. Circle the room until each person has spoken. Include yourself.

What's on top? Ask employees to think about their feelings, situations, plans, or whatever is on their minds. As facilitator, start by sharing "what's on top" for you. Then ask for volunteers. Give everyone a chance to share, if they want to.

Personal interview: Divide your staff into pairs randomly (for example, by counting off). Then distribute sets of questions to be used in mutual interviews, for example:

1. What makes your job easy to do?
2. What makes your job hard to do?
3. List the three most rewarding aspects of your work.
4. Name one big reason why you are good for your job.
5. Name one big reason why your job is good for you.
6. Identify one way you have grown in your job in the last year.
7. Identify one way you would like to grow in your job over the next year.

Ask the pairs to interview each other. Afterward, ask people to rejoin the large group, sitting next to their partners, and to share one or two items they learned about their partners. End by asking people to share their *own* view of one way their partner is good for the organization.

These activities will prove to be gratifying to you and satisfying to your employees.

Strategy 2: Cultivate smooth co-worker relationships. If you view employees as each other's as well as your customers, you need to place as much emphasis on how they treat each other as you do on how they treat the public. The following meeting format is designed to establish guidelines for harmonious co-worker relationships. If you involve your staff in establishing these guidelines, you can secure their commitment to these rules and use the rules to keep people on course in their relationships with co-workers. Introduce the session as a chance to identify behaviors among co-workers that contribute to satisfying relationships.

- Warm people up by asking them to talk about the one thing they wish others really understood about their job or about a model co-worker relationship. Afterward, invite several people to share what they or their partners said with the whole group.
- Now, ask people to think about behaviors of their co-workers that make them feel valued, productive, and supported and the behaviors that make them feel the opposite. Brainstorm two lists.
- Break down into smaller groups to refine and narrow down the list. Each small group must identify the five behaviors that would make a positive difference.
- Reconvene the large group and list all the recommendations. After group discussion consolidate the small-group lists into one list of five behaviors that everyone will adopt to enhance harmonious working relationships. An example is found in the Co-Worker House Rules one group developed:

1. Even if it's not your job, do it or find someone who can.
2. Listen. When someone complains, don't be defensive.
3. Keep co-workers informed. It builds trust and sparks cooperation.
4. Speak to the source of the problem. Talk *to* the person, not behind her or his back.
5. Teamwork. Every person matters. Without every instrument, there is no orchestra.

If you feel you do not have the skills, find someone in your organization who can act as facilitator, perhaps someone from education or staff development or social services or another manager who feels comfortable in this role. These structured, positively oriented activities are not that difficult and you will soon want to try them.

Strategy 3: Learn the language of appreciation and use it. People thirst for recognition and appreciation. You know that. Yet employees frequently report feeling unappreciated. You probably know that too from your own personal experience. At one hospital, in an audit we conducted of the effectiveness of thirty different employee recognition practices, "a pat on the back from my supervisor" won by unanimous vote as most effective practice (compared with merit pay, merchandise awards, certificates, birthday gifts, personal notes from the CEO, and many more).

Why are pats on the back not more frequent? Because you think employees should not be thanked for doing the job they were hired to do? Because if you show appreciation, employees might get cocky and let their performance slip? Because you do not want to play favorites? Because your boss does not appreciate you, so why should you appreciate your employees (lack of role models)?

We daresay that there are two simple keys to increasing employee appreciation. First, stop the excuses and decide to be forthcoming with appreciation, whether your boss is with you or not. Second, become adept at the language of appreciation, so that you do not consume undue time or energy.

If you believe that employees need not be recognized for doing the job they were hired to do, look in the mirror. Do you not want recognition for devoting energy and dedication to the job and not simply toeing the line? If you believe that the recipient of your appreciation may become cocky and slip in performance, think again. Research suggests the opposite, that reinforcement of desired behavior increases the frequency of that desired behavior. You get more of what you want when you reinforce the positive behavior you are already getting.

You do not have to play favorites. Observe all staff members—the stars, the people with problems. You will find positive behavior in every person.

Perhaps your boss does not appreciate you. So take the lead and do what you know is right, whether your boss does it or not. You be the adult in the situation and nurture your employees, instead of blaming others for failing to give your employees this scarce and most precious commodity. Maybe you consistently hold back appreciation to keep your employees striving for your all-too-scarce approval and, thereby, increase your power and control. There is no good excuse for holding back appreciation.

The other obstacle is language. Some people have difficulty expressing their appreciation. They feel awkward and do not know what to say. Learn and then use the following format, over and over. It will not sound redundant because the substance keeps changing.

1. Describe the behavior: "I noticed (or heard) that you worked an extra shift once you realized how short-staffed we were last night."
2. Spell out the consequences (for the customer, the department, the organization, co-workers, and others): "This was a great help to our patients and to your co-workers, who would have been stretched beyond reasonable limits if you hadn't eased their load."
3. Convey empathy: "I realize it's exhausting to work two shifts in a row and it's hard on your family."

4. Express appreciation: "Thank you. I really appreciate it."

As a memory aid, keep this format on a 3 × 5 card at your desk. After lunch, spend a few minutes *planning* statements of appreciation. Then deliver them, face to face or in writing; both methods work.

Strategy 4: Spark a sense of contribution by sharing responsibility for your group's health. Most employees want to influence their work situation. You can help them feel valuable if you share responsibility for the group's health with them. Our staff uses the following format for quarterly meetings. We call it Fix, Bury, Celebrate.

> *Part 1:* Form small groups of three or four at random. Ask them to discuss within their groups how they have been feeling lately about the department (or work group) and then to summarize the results of their discussion in symbols, words, pictures, or whatever. After fifteen minutes, reconvene the entire group and have each small group explain its drawing.
>
> *Part 2:* Break up again into the small groups and make three lists: (1) what we need to *fix*, (2) what we need to *bury* (for example, grudges, old stereotypes), and (3) what we need to *celebrate*. After fifteen minutes, reconvene the large group and share the lists. Compile one grand list that includes items for follow-up and ask for volunteers to work on these items.

Strategy 5: Monitor employee satisfaction and use the results to hold yourself accountable. The focus on fulfilling employee needs must never fade. To hold yourself accountable, institute a method for monitoring, at least bimonthly, employee satisfaction. Then, look at the results. The simple sample survey in Exhibit 4 tracks employee satisfaction on three important factors.

Bimonthly, you can trend the results of the survey on a chart (Figure 6). This regular feedback will alert you to items

Exhibit 4. Employee Satisfaction Survey.

1. How connected do you feel to others in our department?
   not at all 1 2 3 4 very much
2. To what extent do you feel satisfied with your contribution to our department's effectiveness and health?
   not at all 1 2 3 4 very much
3. How recognized and appreciated do you feel at work?
   not at all 1 2 3 4 very much

Figure 6. Trend Chart

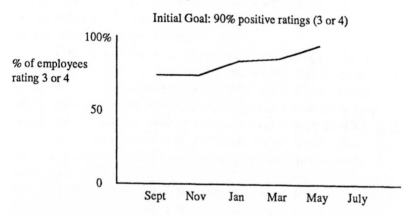

Initial Goal: 90% positive ratings (3 or 4)

requiring attention and improvement. If you are brave and willing to be held accountable, post the results and engage staff in planning get-well action.

When employees are thriving, they have more to give to your organization's customers, and they are committed to giving. By attending to employee needs and supporting them actively in their jobs, you can attract and retain people who will serve the organization's goals with spirit and dedication. You will assemble a group of talented people who unite to face new challenges.

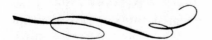

From Reactive to Proactive Behavior

1. Do you usually take on a new project or set a new goal only in response to a request from your boss?　　　　　　　　　　　　YES　NO

2. When problems arise, do you feel relieved after you have put out the fire and can move on to business as usual?　　　　　　　　YES　NO

3. When long-standing problems are made visible do you do nothing because "that's the way it is around here"?　　　　　　　　YES　NO

4. Do you problem-solve only in the face of crisis?　　　　　　　　　　　　　　YES　NO

5. Can you name a disaster waiting to happen within your organization, a disaster that you have not discussed with the people involved?　YES　NO

6. Do you feel too busy to do anything more than handle one crisis after another?　　　YES　NO

7. Do you see yourself as an initiator of new plans and possibilities?　　　　　　　YES　NO

8. Do you have or are you developing a reputation as a go-getter?　　　　　　　　YES　NO

9. Do you occasionally get into trouble for doing things beyond your authority? YES NO
10. Do you voice your opinions on important issues even when nobody asks you? YES NO
11. Are you more likely to make things happen than to observe others making things happen? YES NO
12. Do you discipline yourself to set your own priorities rather than respond to priorities others define for you? YES NO

If you answered "yes" to the first six questions and "no" to the last six questions you probably are more reactive than proactive in your approach to your job. "No" answers to the first six questions and "yes" answers to the last six questions indicate the opposite tendency—to be more proactive than reactive. Reactive managers extinguish one fire after another and are satisfied when they relieve the superficial aspects (symptoms) of a problem. Although such intervention may be effective in the short term, it does little to get to the core of the problem and prevent recurrences.

Reactive managers do not consciously set priorities; instead, they move from crisis to crisis, from deadline to deadline. Initiative is not part of their repertoire; they wait for direction from their superiors, and when such direction is not forthcoming, they complain about the lack of leadership.

Proactive managers are quite different. They anticipate problems and intervene early to prevent them. They think ahead, schedule time for projects important to them, even if these projects fail to attract the attention of others. Unlike reactive managers, they do not feel relieved after quieting a crisis, unless they know how to prevent its recurrence. Reactive managers discuss their questions and concerns with senior management and also with other managers. In short, they take the initiative to solve problems, to make changes, to communicate, to make things happen.

Case 1: Your CEO has announced that the deficit is growing because expenses are skyrocketing. Every manager will have to be part of the solution. Reactive managers most likely wait for the deadline to submit their revised budgets, having produced them in an atmosphere of intense pressure. Proactive managers are more likely to begin immediately to analyze expenses and prepare cost reduction plans, so that they can submit a carefully revised budget on short notice.

Case 2: Hospitals *magazine reports that JCAHO has decided to shift from use of process indicators to outcome indicators in accreditation of hospitals. Although some key clinical indicators have already been identified, JCAHO is spearheading studies of other possible indicators of hospital quality. This will apply to every department in the organization.* Reactive managers hear this news and do nothing until they are forced to. On the other hand, proactive managers investigate this new JCAHO direction, learn all they can about it, and think how they might institute outcome measurement in their departments; if outcome measurement is inevitable, is it not wise to get a jump on the new system?

Case 3: Doctor Hesperus is angry and calls you, the director of pharmacy, to complain that your pharmacy is short-staffed at night when he needs medication orders filled quickly. Reactive managers talk with Doctor Hesperus and attempt to calm him, explaining the realities that make short staffing at night unavoidable. Proactive managers reconsider the situation to determine whether the short staffing is having serious consequences not only for Dr. Hesperus's patients but also for others. They poll other physicians and staff to determine the extent of the limited service. And, if they find that staff must be increased, they do the analytical work necessary to acquire additional resources.

Case 4: You have several tasks of equal importance. Your administrator says, "Do them all!" but you know it is impossible to do them all well. Reactive managers let the tougher, long-term tasks slide, hoping the boss will be too busy to notice. Or they ask the boss to prioritize the tasks for them. Proactive managers are more likely to examine the possibilities, select those they believe are most important, act on them, and inform the boss in their next routine report.

Benefits of Proactive Behavior Versus Reactive Behavior

In a recent strategic planning retreat with a vibrant and enterprising executive team in a large teaching hospital, the CEO lamented, "We're so good at handling crises, but it's so tiring. I just wish we could *avert* disasters waiting to happen." One vice-president suggested, "Let's identify those disasters that we know will happen if we don't do anything now to prevent them." The group identified several potential disasters, which they believed would occur within the next six months and would be highly destructive to the organization. They joked that if they successfully averted the disasters, they would be eliminating their chance to respond and enjoy the satisfaction gained from resolution of a crisis. And, others would not credit them for effective intervention. Prevention of a crisis is an invisible accomplishment.

The disadvantages of proactive management make reactive management even more attractive. Prevention of a problem requires self-discipline; you must allocate time to work on a problem that does not appear to be very important, yet. Proactive management seems more methodical than exciting. You control the pace; there is no crisis compelling you to act. Also, when you manage proactively, you stick your neck out.

Nevertheless, proactive management reaps clear personal benefits for those managers who embrace it:

- When you act to prevent problems, instead of handling them one by one, you do not have to fight the same fires year in and year out. This releases your energy for other things.
- Others respect initiative; they respect you as a leader and change maker. You are seen as a key player, not a finger pointer.
- Proactive management is healthier. When you are reactive, you live in a permanent state of anxiety as you wonder what you are going to have to deal with next.

From reactive to proactive: both ends of the continuum have costs and benefits for the manager, but the configuration of costs and benefits for the organization has changed.

Health care cultures of the past accepted and reinforced reactivity in managers. If the organization were rolling along smoothly, making ends meet, and avoiding public scrutiny, there was little impetus to do more than attend to erupting crises. In stable, financially sound organizations, the motivation to operate proactively did not exist.

Now, however, a reactive, troubleshooting style of management has obvious negative consequences for the organization—consequences that are dramatic and cumulative. Recurring problems interfere with patient, physician, and staff satisfaction. The hospital down the street that has found ways to eliminate such problems can satisfy its customers and yours better than you can. So consumer choice and loyalty and the hospital's reputation and revenue are affected. In the face of increasing resource constraints, high productivity and efficiency are business necessities but are impossible to achieve when recurrent problems consume all your energy. In a lean and mean environment, you do not have the slack to drop everything and work on crises.

Because the new economic climate increases the pressure placed on staff, you must be concerned with the effect on morale. People run out of steam fast in a crisis management environment. Staff may also begin to question their manager's competence when they see the same crises recur time and time again. They wonder why no one takes action to prevent these crises.

Reactive management maintains equilibrium. Today, however, equilibrium must give way to deliberate and continuous improvement. Executives must focus on advancing relationships between the organization and the external environment and on building an overall business strategy. You must move the organization forward—from the inside out—with leadership and foresight. Proactive management is a must.

To push yourself toward a more consistent proactive

stance, read avidly in your professional field; stay abreast of developments. Attend professional meetings to expand your understanding of trends and issues and to make new contacts. When you think an issue should be addressed, raise it. When you think a decision should be questioned, question it. When you have an idea, advance it. At least weekly, review priorities for the next week, month, and year. Act on them and modify them as needed. Push yourself to identify potential disasters and take steps to prevent them. Think through your work routines. Note the different types of problems you would like to solve, for example, people problems, resource-utilization problems, cumbersome procedure problems, staff morale problems, interdepartmental problems, and patterns of customer complaints. Target two or three to tackle before anyone tells you to do so.

Strategies That Foster Proactive Behavior

Four strategies can help you escape the reactive management cycle and become proactive: (1) Free up your time for proaction. (2) Take initiative in increments. (3) Do your homework. (4) Engage in energizing self-talk.

Strategy 1: Free up your time for proaction. Many managers want to be proactive but say they do not have the time. To move from a reactive to a proactive style, these managers need to rethink how they spend their time. When they do so, this excuse loses its validity. Does this situation sound familiar?

> I can't believe the things I spend my time on. I hire people who I think are good people. Then, I seem to end up doing their jobs for them.
>
> Just yesterday, one of my managers said, "I'm not sure how to do this." The job is tough and I figured I could do it myself quicker than I could explain it to him. Then, another person on my staff said she had to leave early and couldn't finish a certain report. Because the dead-

line was upon us and I was the one responsible for turning that report in on time, and because this employee was owed the time off, I took the report half-done and had to stop what I was doing to finish it. Then, another employee stopped in to complain about another department not giving him some information he needed, so I called that other department to put the pressure on.

To make a long story short, my day was gone—eaten away by things I didn't expect to have to do and things that I felt I shouldn't be doing. When I got to work that morning, I had big plans about taking a look at a problem that's been bugging all of us. That would have been proactive. But then, I ended up doing what one employee didn't know how to do, finishing another's report so she could leave early, and getting into a fray with another department to get information for one of my staff, so he could simply do what I asked of him. My day was gone!

On the way home, I felt annoyed with myself for getting nowhere on my priorities and I felt furious at my staff for giving me their work and expecting me to fight their battles.

Many managers express similar frustration and claim that they would be proactive if they had the time.

Perhaps you too feel that you cannot carry more "baggage" than you already are. Let us examine the baggage analogy further. Your staff's responsibilities are their baggage. Saddled with this baggage, staff respond in various ways:

- It's too heavy. Can you grab one end of it?
- This isn't my baggage. Will you please take it and find the person it belongs to?
- I have more than I can carry already. Can't you please find someone else to carry it?

- I've never carried baggage quite like this before and I don't think I know exactly how to carry it.
- I'm so busy just now. Can you just hang onto this for me until I can see my way clear to carry it?
- I realize you need this tomorrow at noon in order to catch your plane, but I just won't be able to get it to you in time. If you want it then, you'd better take it yourself now.
- You asked for this now and here it is, but I didn't have enough time so I might have left out a few necessities.

In so many situations, managers take the baggage from the employee because they feel responsible; however, they end up feeling overburdened.

If you really are too busy to be proactive, you are carrying too many bags or the wrong bags. You have to relieve your burden and free up time for proactive efforts, possibly through the following approaches.

Stop being so willing to carry your employees' baggage. Make them carry their own. Schedule thirty-minute meetings weekly with each person you supervise to review their responsibilities and make sure they are clear on what they need to do. At this meeting, identify the responsibilities the employee wants to unload on you and discuss how the employee, not you, can walk out of the room and fulfill those responsibilities. Make it clear: "I consider this to be your responsibility [your problem to solve, your project to move on]. How can we in the next few minutes prepare you to do what needs to be done?" Resist the temptation to take over when staff members express confusion or insecurity, even if intervention will make you feel brilliant and needed.

If your staff cannot develop the muscles needed to carry their own baggage, find staff who can.

Pack only as many bags as your people can manage and you can monitor. Otherwise, bags will be lost and you will waste time trying to find them.

Discuss the responsibilities face-to-face or on the phone. If you communicate only in writing, you will not know whether your employees grasp their responsibilities.

We are talking about delegation, leveraging your own power through effective use of your staff. If you make delegation a priority, you will create the time needed to manage proactively.

Strategy 2: Take initiative in increments. To be proactive, you must take initiative. The continuum from reactivity to initiative includes six steps:

1. Do nothing; resist action even when asked to act.
2. Await instructions and then act accordingly.
3. Ask for instructions.
4. Suggest what you might do and, if agreed upon, do it.
5. Take action on your own but tell others (your boss and other key players) immediately.
6. Take action on your own and tell others as you routinely update them on your activities.

Steps 1, 2, and 3 are reactive modes. Proaction begins at Step 4 and peaks at Step 6.

In one community hospital in the upper Midwest, six managers shared their frustration with the slowness of change in their organization. Many systems and quality problems simply were not addressed. They decided to form a breakfast club. They met weekly at 7 A.M. to formulate strategies for making the changes needed in the organization. No one had asked them to do so. They did this because they decided it was important. They implemented the solutions to some problems. They recommended solutions to other problems to the executive team. These managers assumed responsibility for progress and problem solving.

Assess your current position on the continuum and begin consciously and deliberately to work your way toward proactive management by taking initiative in increments to minimize anxiety and risk.

Strategy 3: Do your homework. Said one director of

pharmacy in a large East Coast hospital, "Being proactive is fine in theory. But when you initiate what you think is a great idea and it gets shot down without a thorough hearing, you learn to keep your ideas to yourself."

This manager and many like her can point to several instances where they took the initiative and were thwarted by the executive team.

Maybe this manager did propose a great idea but was met with closedmindedness and instant rejection. Consider the possibility that she failed to do what was necessary to ensure a fair and thorough hearing. One administrator describes a case in point.

> I asked my department heads to come up with new ideas and proposals. I said, we need to become more innovative. One of my department heads came to me excited about launching an ambitious community education program sponsored by our hospital. Since we have done only fragmented programs in the past, I was initially enthusiastic. I said, "Sounds promising. I'd like to hear more about what you envision. Between now and our next meeting, how about spelling out what this kind of program would look like." She agreed.
>
> At our next meeting, she showed me a proposed curriculum that showed an array of program titles and who in our organization might conduct them. I looked it over and said that the offerings sounded good, but that I needed to know much more before making a decision. I had to know the costs involved and the potential revenue, how we would promote the programs, who would run them, how we would choose doctors as speakers without alienating doctors we didn't choose, and so on. I asked her to go back and work out the details. She never did. When I asked her about it later, she said she gave up because I wasn't enthusiastic.

How can these managers expect us to
approve of their ideas if they haven't done their
homework on them. When we ask them to do
their homework, they take it as rejection and
blame us for discouraging their initiative. I'm
not squelching their initiative. All I want is a
complete plan, not a lazy, thrown together proposal that I myself have to finish in order to evaluate it.

If you need executive approval for plans or ideas, you
need to go further than the idea stage to sell your idea. You
need to anticipate questions, obstacles, and problems and
evaluate costs and benefits for the organization in thorough
detail. If you do not think it through, you are doing little
more than delegating upward to a busy administrator. If you
want to make that vision a reality, do your homework and
you will be in a markedly stronger position to "sell" your
idea to your boss.

Develop the idea into a full-scale proposal, complete
with plans, needed resources, an evaluation of costs and benefits, and implementation strategy. If you have the authority
to move on it, do so with the confidence that it is well conceived. If you need approval, you can now sell it more effectively to the powers that be.

Use this blueprint to make your vision a reality:

Blueprint for Making Your Case

1. Clarify your goal(s).
2. Identify your reasons, for customers, your department,
   the organization, and so on.
3. Identify the key people or groups whose support you
   need.
4. Anticipate the reasons they might resist and plan to
   address these. Determine in great detail the costs and risks
   involved. Show that you have thought through everything carefully and are not proceeding blindly.

5. Spell out in great detail all possible benefits for you, your staff, your department, the administration, your boss in particular, the organization, and your organization's customers. Obtain or project numbers to document these benefits. Compare future benefits with past statistics.
6. Now put it all together. Articulate your case so that the decision makers are convinced they cannot live without your idea.
7. Remain confident and assertive. Expect the people you address to realize that you are making sense and to support the proposal. If they do not support it, act surprised. Persist. If you still get a "no" but remain convinced that the organization is making a big mistake, find support among other opinion leaders, build a committee, do not give up.

If you want to be proactive, you must work hard, but you will be gratified by the results.

Strategy 4: Engage in energizing self-talk. The other tactic that can help you move from a reactive to a proactive management style is internal. It involves your personal thoughts or self-talk. When you recognize a problem, do you think "that's not my problem," "that's been here forever and it will outlive me," "I'm not going to care until someone else does," or "why bother?"

In Chapter One, we described the "thought-feeling-action" triangle, claiming that you can change your feelings and actions by altering your thoughts. When problems or opportunities arise, tell yourself what to do or not do. This self-talk affects your feelings and your inclination to behave proactively versus reactively.

If you want to move toward the proactive end of the continuum, examine your self-talk and modify it so that it pushes you toward that goal. This means recognizing the self-talk that keeps you passive and replacing it with self-talk that spurs you into action.

Middle managers have shared with us the changes they made in their self-talk to become more proactive:

I used to think:	*Now, I choose to think:*
If it isn't broken, don't fix it.	If it isn't broken, maybe I haven't looked hard enough.
That's not my problem. I'll act when I have to.	I'm responsible. Act now. Don't wait.
Later maybe.	Get off the dime and do it now.
If I act, I'll be too visible.	If I don't act, I'll be dispensable.

To help yourself become more proactive, determine what self-talk stops you from taking initiative and record it in writing. Now, substitute each hindering thought with a thought that spurs you to act. Read these new self-statements fifty times. With increasing passion, say them aloud to a friend. Write the most effective lines on an index card, and keep the card on the corner of your desk. Read it daily to ingrain these thoughts in your mind.

The proactive manager's motto is, If it is to be, it is up to me. It is my responsibility.

In our rapidly changing environment, you must make rapid and pervasive changes simply to keep up, let alone get ahead. It would be nice if there were a director of initiative whose job it was to take the initiative necessary to move your organization forward. But such a person could not make enough happen fast enough. Each manager has to identify and tackle problems and seize opportunities on his or her own. Managers at every level must lead the organization forward with their collective strength and talent.

In summary, to move from a reactive to a proactive style of management, know what you want, know how to get it, do the work involved, believe in yourself, and talk yourself into action.

From Tradition and Safety to Experimentation and Risk

1. Do you habitually search for new and better approaches to your work?   YES   NO
2. Do you ask a lot of questions, without worrying about whether they reveal your ignorance?   YES   NO
3. Does your desire to make things work better take up at least as much time as your working to maintain them the way they are?   YES   NO
4. Do you feel excited about your work?   YES   NO
5. Do you sometimes try a new method even if you are not sure it will work?   YES   NO
6. Do you think of new ideas on your way to work or in the shower?   YES   NO
7. Do you deal with mistakes and failures as learning experiences?   YES   NO
8. Do you feel uncomfortable when open discussion and disagreements occur among your staff?   YES   NO
9. Do you find yourself asking for permission before you try something new?   YES   NO
10. Do you receive new ideas with skepticism rather than enthusiasm?   YES   NO

103

11. Do you have a hard time letting go of past
    mistakes and forgiving yourself?   YES NO
12. Do you avoid doing things that are new or
    unfamiliar?   YES NO
13. Do you find yourself resisting other people's
    ideas and suggestions before you have really
    entertained them?   YES NO
14. Do you hesitate to disagree with others for
    fear of alienating them or losing their
    approval?   YES NO

"Yes" answers to the first seven questions and "no"
answers to the last seven questions reflect an inclination
toward experimentation and risk, rather than toward tradition
and safety. Tradition- and safety-oriented managers prefer the
status quo and a stable and secure workplace. Managers
inclined toward experimentation and risk prefer challenge
and novelty.

Tradition, Safety, Sameness

"We're part of a long, proud medical tradition." Does that
line not trigger a sense of pride and altruism in you? We are,
after all, in an industry with caring at its heart. And medicine
and medical care cultures have developed traditions that make
us proud, perhaps blindly proud. Underneath, we have tied
ourselves unquestioningly to past practices, whether they still
serve our interests or not. We have worshipped and glorified
our traditions so much so that we now have trouble differ-
entiating between those that work and those that do not.
Change and experimentation are very sensitive, even political,
issues because so many health care professionals interpret
them as rejections of the hallowed traditions of the past.

As you well know, however, not all of our traditions
are helpful, for example, long waits for patients, friction and
disrespect between physicians and nurses, sharply demarcated
turf lines between departments that cannot be crossed even to

solve mutual problems, lost charts, and billing errors. These are all traditions!

Imagine that you are in a meeting with colleagues. Another colleague walks into the room and trips on a coat rack that protrudes in front of the door. Your colleague stands the coat rack back up and sits down at the table to join the meeting. A few minutes later, another colleague arrives late for the meeting. This person also walks in, falls over the coat rack, and stands it back in place. A few minutes later, yet another colleague enters and does the same thing. Would it not make sense for someone to move the coat rack to another part of the room, away from the door?

In many hospitals, patients and staff run into the same impediments time and again, but instead of removing the impediment, we view it as simply the way things are done here.

Before prospective payment, before competition, before the nursing shortage, before the technology revolution, before consumer scrutiny, our organizations could focus on maintenance of quality and preservation of the delicate balance among the complex systems, jobs, procedures, and forces. The manager's job was to keep their people and systems on course.

New managers, enthusiastic and ready to make their mark by instituting change quickly, learned to moderate this enthusiasm and abide by tradition. Managers who questioned tradition and persisted in their advocacy of change were likely to be labeled as mavericks, a label with a negative connotation to those determined to protect long-held practices.

These dynamics were a product of the times. Health care organizations prided themselves on stability, solidity, and unflagging reliability. Being charged with caring for the sick and vulnerable, we took pains to develop predictable, secure systems. Safety has been a driving force because we take very seriously our responsibility for people's lives. A system driven to ensure safety and security inevitably strives toward predictable, routine operations.

Not too different from the dynamics that developed in Detroit's auto industry. The United States maintained an edge over foreign car manufacturers for many years. European manufacturers lost competitive time when they had to rebuild their factories as a result of wartime destruction. Then, Asian producers entered the American marketplace with unforeseen horsepower. Meanwhile, U.S. producers reveled in their success. Investment in innovation, serious research and development, and significant changes dampened short-term profits and received low priority. Complacency in the face of success pervaded until Chrysler went public with its failures and dramatized the need to rebuild and focus on innovation and continuous improvement.

Similarly in health care, managers who believe that our systems and procedures have worked for years and will continue to do so are dangerous. Our systems and practices sorely need revitalization. And this cannot happen without deliberate, focused experimentation spearheaded by managers.

We are going through time compression in health care. What used to take a decade to evolve has gradually been reduced to six months. Therefore, adherence to past practices, without question, no longer suffices. The only practice that should now be a constant is accommodation to change. The sign over the door should read: "Subject to change on short notice." To be resilient in the face of externally imposed change, an experimenting, flexible approach is key. Our strength lies in our capacity to learn and adapt quickly.

Consider burgeoning technology. Although breakthroughs are exciting, they wreak havoc with our current delivery systems. Previous inpatient services are now outpatient services. Procedures that required many staff now require one technologist and a fancy machine. Entirely new diagnostic procedures need a home and a delivery system that matches the appropriate patients to them. And more.

There has been a tendency to patch up our systems and tax them to the limit to absorb new technology. But the limit has been reached. We can put only so many Band-Aids on our scheduling systems, computer systems, staffing patterns, service units, reimbursement mechanisms, and delivery methods.

We need to make some very deep and wrenching changes instead of patching up or overextending the old, unsuitable methods. We must instigate change and, instead of lamenting, embrace it with energy and excitement.

If you are not moving forward, you are probably backsliding relative to your competition. As manager, you have several options: (1) You can watch what is happening. (2) You can make things happen. (3) You can wonder what happened. Option 2 is a necessity.

At one large teaching hospital, department directors complained about red tape involved in making the purchases required to run their departments. Delays and lost paperwork were the norm. One group of frustrated department directors decided to track the purchasing process and identify the snags. They started by examining the five-part purchasing form. To learn how the form proceeded through the system, they assigned five people to the five parts of the form. As each part of the form proceeded through the hospital's complex system, the accompanying person also went along, from department to department, desk to desk.

To make a long story short, this investigative team discovered that only three of the five copies were of any real value. The other two copies caused delays and problems but did not trigger a single necessary action. These copies had become obsolete, but nobody had revamped the form because it had been done that way for years.

Sound unbelievable? Ask yourself: What systems and processes in your organization have taken on a life of their own, causing problems and delays that people throughout the organization have learned to live with? You probably can generate quite a long list. It is not surprising. We make rules and design methods for reasons that make good sense. We follow these rules and adhere to these methods. Time passes and conditions change. Although the once sound reasons for our rules and methods no longer exist, the rules remain in place. We become conditioned and fail to think or take responsibility for our actions.

The Manager's Role

If your organization is like most others in health care, the systems, processes, products, and supplies are so complex that no one person or no one department can detect and solve all the problems. The only hope is for you, the manager, to include in your role the function of obsolescence detector and innovator.

In this environment, you cannot adhere to traditions with security and stability as their only justification. Instead, you must adopt a mindset that supports experimentation and risk. Managers at every level must be willing to stick their necks out to do away with outmoded practices and pave new paths.

You are faced with a continuum from enslavement by tradition on one end to experimentation on the other end. The tradition-bound, safety-oriented manager:

• Thinks "This is the way things are" rather than "Here's how things could be"
• Says "We can't," not "How can we?"
• Justifies current practices by explaining how long the organization has sustained them
• Relies heavily on received wisdom when faced with decisions
• Feels uncomfortable with the concept of risk and can cite many reasons why it should be avoided for the sake of the organization
• May resist making changes because they do not coincide with the job description

On the other hand, the experimenting, risk-taking manager:

• Welcomes new ideas and possibilities
• Says "How can we?" before "We can't"
• Shows a willingness to move beyond received wisdom and think for oneself
• Views missteps and failures as learning experiences

- Works to sustain a high batting average, not perfection, to feel free to take risks
- Recognizes that new ways are inherently experiments and will not always work
- Does not dwell on the discrepancy between the original job description and what is now being asked

Case 1: You see a need to revamp your scheduling system to shorten the length of patient waiting time. You know that you must involve certain key physicians whose personal schedules would be affected. Tradition-bound managers do nothing for fear of making waves, or go to their superiors for permission to move on this idea, thereby eliminating their risk. Experimenting managers are more likely to make plans to move ahead because they assume they have the latitude to act. They talk with the physicians involved and develop a plan. They do not ask permission, but they do keep their superiors informed of their actions.

Case 2: You have been asked by your boss to reexamine one of your department's practices to see whether there might be a way to increase efficiency. You raise the question at a meeting with your staff. The people who speak up claim that the current method is the most efficient and nothing would be gained by changing it. The tradition-bound manager listens carefully and probes for a solid rationale for continuing current practices that he or she can convey to the boss. The experimenting manager pushes staff to set aside current practices and envision refinements. Such managers know there are always better ways.

Case 3: You have a bright idea and you move ahead to implement it. Upon hearing your idea, a colleague warns you about sticking your neck out and tells you that you are crazy to try and change things. The tradition-bound manager rethinks the soundness of his or her intentions and succumbs to the "why risk it" atmosphere. The experimenting manager is more likely to thank the colleague for the opinion, admit that it might prove true, and persist in the plan to move ahead, purporting "nothing ventured, nothing gained." And, secretly, he or she is flattered and delighted to be perceived as a maverick.

Case 4: You have developed what you believe is a better way to perform one of your department's key functions. You have mapped out a trial run and involved your staff in its implementation. The idea creates more problems than it solves. After such an experience, tradition-bound, risk-averse managers avoid any other departures from tradition; however, experimenting, risk-taking managers focus on what they learned from the failure and devise a new experiment. In discussing the failure with staff, they are positive and emphasize what was learned and how it can be used to guide further problem solving. They reinforce that "You can't move forward unless you stick your neck out."

Case 5: Your boss has encouraged managers throughout your organization to become innovative and experimental. You took this message seriously. You tried a new "solution" to a long-standing problem and your solution did not work. Your boss expresses disappointment in you for this failure. Experimenting, risk-taking managers do not apologize. They tactfully confront their boss's response as discrepant with his or her espoused values, as in this example:

> You asked us to experiment and take risks. I did. Although I did what I could to minimize the risk involved by planning carefully, the experiment failed. By being angry at me for having tried, you are discouraging me from the experimentation and risk taking in which you want us to engage. What *do* you want from me? If you want me to experiment with new and better ways, some of my efforts will inevitably fail and I will learn from them. If you want to encourage experimentation, it does not help to slap my hand when one effort fails.

Self-renewing, experimenting managers succeed and fail, take criticism and grow. They know life has many chapters!

The Personal Costs and Benefits

Why do health care people not depart more often from tradition and take more risks? In our discussions, managers repeatedly cite ten benefits of sustaining tradition and avoiding experimentation and risk:

- You can blame tradition and your managerial ancestors when things do not work.
- You know what to expect and do not have to handle surprises. The known feels a whole lot safer than the unknown.
- You do not have to explain the way you do things if you do them the way they have always been done. You only have to justify departures from tradition.
- When you follow tradition, you can fade into the woodwork, avoiding the scrutiny of onlookers.
- When you support things as they are, you do not have to make new demands on other people.
- Risk takers are seen by some people as organizational irritants. If the risk takers are few, they might feel isolated and even a little crazy.
- When you experiment, you do not know every outcome, so you cannot reassure others or keep promises.
- It can be anxiety provoking to live with the uncertainty inherent in experimentation and risk taking.
- You might need new skills to pull off your plans.
- You will have to deal with flack when experiments do not work.

No wonder so many managers hesitate to become experimenters and risk takers! But consider the other side—the ben-

efits of experimentation and risk reported by managers who
have successfully made a transition:

- A prominent cause of stress and burnout is
  boredom. Experimentation and risk can be
  exciting—an adventure.
- When you always do what you always did, you
  always get what you always got. If you want
  more than that, you have a problem.
- When you experiment, you see improvements,
  not the same old problems.
- You and your peers hold you in higher esteem;
  you are viewed as a mover and shaker, not a
  drone.
- Experimentation and the adventure involved
  in it are contagious. Your staff catches it.
- You are bound to succeed some of the time
  and victories are satisfying.
- In today's business climate, the innovative,
  risk-taking manager is more marketable, more
  promotable, and more likely to attract executive attention.

Obviously there are risks associated with the shift to
experimentation and risk taking, but the benefits are increasing in the current environment where the status quo no
longer suffices.

Strategies That Boost Experimentation and Risk

We hope you are convinced that experimentation and risk
taking are worth nurturing, that you have much to gain personally and professionally from increasing your own comfort
with and inclinations in that direction. Exercise your personal power, test your limits, and accept nothing less than
optimal results. Playing it safe is comforting, but you get
into deeper and deeper ruts and eventually a grave.

From our work with organizations in transition, we

have identified strategies that help managers build the muscle and confidence needed to experiment and take risks. Take stock of your attitudes and skills, and seek those strategies you can use to help yourself change: (1) Adopt an "experimenter mindset." (2) Exercise your creative muscles. (3) Engage in intelligent risk taking; calculate and lessen your risk. (4) Cultivate allies. (5) Lavish attention on experiments and on the people who have the guts to engage in them.

   Strategy 1: Adopt an "experimenter mindset." A manager with an experimenter mindset tests hypotheses much like a scientist does, believing that improvement is always possible. He or she analyzes a problem and determines which option would most likely reap the desired results. After implementation, the experimenting manager examines whether the results match expectations. If so, the experiment is successful. If the results are disappointing, he or she concludes that the hypothesis failed and seeks to learn why, searching for a new hypothesis that is more likely to work. The experimenter does not expect 100 percent success, does not expect to find panaceas, does not take failure personally, and does not fall apart in the wake of occasional disapproval.

   For many of us in health care, these attitudes do not come easy. The experimenter may not expect 100 percent success; however, in many health care cultures, failure is not tolerated. As a result, managers hesitate to "try" unless success is ensured.

   In health care, we hesitate to call a solution a solution unless it solves the problem 100 percent. But, can you think of one significant problem in your organization that has a 100 percent solution? In most cases, the best we can hope for in this superspecialized complex we call a health care organization are partial solutions and incremental improvements. The experimenter may not take failure personally, but how many managers feel comfortable with a "You win some, you lose some" attitude? Although the experimenter may maintain confidence in the wake of disapproval after a failed experiment, many of us feel hurt and do not persist in our commitment to change.

To emulate the experimenter and adopt an experimenter mindset, we need to distance ourselves as individuals from the outcomes of our experiments. That is, we need to develop a thicker skin. And we need to believe that improvement is always possible; it is simply a matter of persistence and a positive attitude.

See failure as a chance to learn: Our self-talk has a great impact here. After trying and failing, many people view themselves as failures. No wonder, they hesitate to try again. Instead, they should be proud that they acted boldly and should learn from both positive and negative results.

Thicken your skin. When your hands are slapped for a failed experiment (and they will be unless you are perfect), live and learn.

Believe in the possibilities. Resist the temptation to view tasks as impossible. The idea for the Pennsylvania Turnpike was termed "Governor Earle's folly." People insisted that cars could not be built to withstand the constant high speeds the road encouraged. Many years ago, British surgeon Stephen Paget declared, "Surgery of the heart has probably reached the limits set by nature. . . . No new method and no new discovery can overcome the natural difficulties that attend a wound of the heart." According to past theories of aerodynamics, the bumblebee cannot fly. Fortunately, the bumblebee is ignorant of this simple truth. We have walked on the moon, immunized millions against measles, created imaging processes, cured many cancers, and much more. We should certainly be able to run health care organizations. Right? Whatever we think is impossible is not necessarily.

If you want to become an experimenter, identify thoughts that discourage experimentation and replace them with thoughts that spur action.

No	Yes
I blew it.	Live and learn.
That's impossible.	The question is how?
I'm sorry. Never again.	Nothing ventured, nothing gained.

| I've survived this long this way. It has always worked before. | There's more to life than survival and I want it. A new day demands new solutions. |

Thomas Watson, founder of IBM, advises, "The way to succeed is to double your failure rate."

Strategy 2: Exercise your creative muscles. Once you accept the need to experiment, you must generate new ideas by switching your perspective. Consider two approaches: (1) Remove self-imposed blocks on your own creativity. (2) Develop your ability to think divergently.

Are you your own worst enemy when it comes to creativity? Do you engage in self-talk that slows your ability to generate new ideas and solutions? Do these phrases ring a bell? Never in a million years. Yes, but . . . We tried that. I'm not creative. It might not work. Such self-talk impedes creativity and experimentation. Replace these phrases with positive thoughts: I'm creative. The more offbeat the better. It will loosen me up.

Consider your capacity to think divergently. Many managers have finely tuned planning skills that they integrate into a cycle like that in Figure 7. Such a linear process helps managers to control their areas of operation. Experimentation and innovation, however, necessitate a process that has been empirically found to be less linear. Pinchot (1985, p. 18) advocates the innovation process illustrated in Figure 8, which involves divergent, creative thinking.

Figure 7. Traditional Planning Cycle.

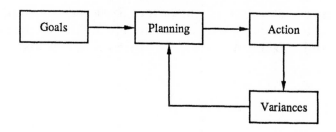

Figure 8. The Innovation Process.

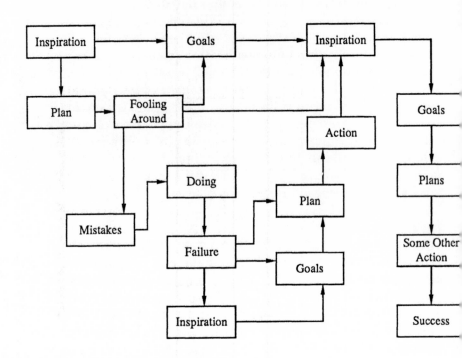

To generate experiments worthy of effort, you need to loosen your thinking and tone up your creative muscles, muscles that can atrophy as a result of disuse. You might benefit from an exercise program. Resources (books, professional seminars) to help you cultivate your creativity are abundant. We present here four techniques that have proven helpful with health care managers in particular: (1) "what iffing," (2) tradition burials, (3) formal experiments, (4) ten-minute improvement meetings. Try them alone and with your staff to fertilize divergent thinking and trigger fresh perspectives on everyday situations, problems, and opportunities.

Permit yourself to suspend the constraints that stifle you in generating ideas. For instance, imagine that a fire destroyed your department's physical facilities. No one was hurt. Now you are part of a team formed to design the new department. What would you build into the design to improve it dramatically? If you had absolutely no financial constraints, what other features would you add?

After "what iffing," one can usually identify improvements that are possible with the existing resources.

Establish a "what if question of the week" program to trigger creative muscle building. Note these examples: What if we treated every patient as we would want our mothers treated? What if we felt no hesitation about confronting managers of other departments who do not support this department? What if we had exactly half the time we now have to serve our customers? What if we lost our policy and procedure manual? What if we received five personal computers as a gift?

If your staff are wedded to tradition, point out a few traditions that do not seem to work anymore. List these on a sheet of paper or chalkboard for all to see. Hold a burial ceremony for those that wreak havoc with effectiveness and customer satisfaction, complete with sentimental eulogy. This can help you and your staff grieve over the loss of these sacred cows and move on to generate improvements.

Challenge staff to join one of several experiments you have designed to test alternative solutions to a problem.

Ideally, engage staff in generating the alternatives and facilitate the formation of teams that develop and debug the plan as well as take responsibility for its implementation. Schedule a future meeting at which the results can be reported. Consider setting up a discretionary fund so that staff teams can apply for seed money for their experiments. Some departments allocate $1000 per year, which is often adequate to encourage experimental thinking.

Expect staff to generate ideas for improvement and provide a structure that sparks their thinking. Use the following staff meeting format for this purpose:

1. Divide your staff into groups of three.
2. Define the task: To generate a better way to do *anything* in the department, to solve any problem or enhance any aspect of service, no matter how large or small.
3. Have each group select a note taker. Set a specific time limit (for example, twenty minutes), after which you reconvene the whole group.
4. Invite each trio to share their results. Ask listeners to refrain from making skeptical comments. Then, after all persons have *quickly* shared their solutions, review each solution and decide on the next move. Should the solution be implemented by one person, debugged by a committee, or handled in some other manner? If ideas are not translated into action, your staff will not be willing to devote energy to innovation and problem solving.

Designate a regular time during staff meetings when you will tackle small problems or generate ideas to be considered further by ad hoc teams.

Strategy 3: Engage in intelligent risk taking; calculate and lessen your risk. If you consciously and conscientiously attend to the snags or loopholes before implementation, you can minimize or eliminate most sources of risk. Think through your experiment ahead of time, anticipate the contingencies at each step, and troubleshoot.

One approach that will improve your batting average

we call solution analysis. With solution analysis, you use a set of questions to help you debug your plan before implementation:

- Think of as many obstacles to success as you can. Be paranoid.
- For each obstacle, rate on a scale from 0 to 4, the likelihood of occurrence and the seriousness. Multiply the two ratings to determine the priority of this obstacle.
- Starting with the highest-priority obstacle, determine causes and contributing factors.
- Generate *preventive* actions: For the main causes, identify actions that will prevent the obstacle from occurring or limit the damage incurred.
- Generate *reactive* strategies. Imagine that you have failed to avoid the obstacles and picture the most likely consequences. Devise actions you can take to minimize the damage. If you can take action to minimize damage, you reduce the seriousness of the obstacle.
- Incorporate the preceding actions into your overall plan now, before the damage is done.

You can use a chart (Exhibit 5) to guide analysis.

Another risk-reducing strategy is the trial run. Trial runs are common sense; they minimize failures and disappointments. But many managers avoid them because they take time and require patience. In a trial run you test your ideas and evaluate their effectiveness in reaching your objective *before* you stick your neck out very far. Ask yourself the following questions:

- Can I try out this idea on people whose opinions I trust (a friend, a peer)?
- Can I form a focus group with the intended beneficiaries of this idea to seek their opinions? For instance, one administrator wanted to institute an employee recognition system. Both she and others on the administrative team thought it was a terrific idea. She scheduled a one-hour

Exhibit 5. Plan for Minimizing Risk.

Desired Result:

Summary of Strategy:

Scale
0 = Not at all
1 = Not very
2 = Moderately
3 = Very
4 = Extremely

What Might Go Wrong	How Likely	How Serious	Priority	Contributory Factors or Causes	Preventive Actions	By Whom	When	Actions that Minimize the Effects	By Whom	When
	×	=								
	×	=								
	×	=								
	×	=								
	×	=								
	×	=								

discussion with employees representative of the target group of the recognition system. They thought the idea was quite misguided. Had she implemented her terrific idea, she surely would have obtained negative results. The trial run minimized her risk.

- Can I implement this idea on a limited scale first? I can work with a small group or department now and, if successful, extend implementation throughout the organization.
- Can I simulate the experiment before implementing it? Especially for changes in procedure, you can usually assemble a group to role-play the key people affected by the proposed change.
- Can I collect data on results before I have to make the "go" or "no-go" decision? Once you do implement, decide in advance on the length of the trial period. Let people know it is an experiment and that you will use the results, for instance after three months, to decide whether to extend implementation.

Strategy 4: Cultivate allies. There is safety in numbers. If your superiors do not support experimentation and risk taking and you are extremely fearful about sticking your neck out, find allies. Identify other people in the organization who stand to benefit from the experiment or who you think would appreciate your effort. Sell your idea to them and assertively solicit their support. Most people will be flattered and respond positively, even though you might not expect them to. You can present your plans or defend them as a group, whose members are united in mutual support.

We have been told that such mutual support is commonplace, but not around positive projects. Managers admit that alliances form around people's cynical perceptions of senior management and around all the reasons why experimentation is unwise. People support each other in making excuses for trying nothing new. Managers admit that to unite behind projects and advocate them as a group would be a bold, tantalizing move.

Strategy 5: Lavish attention on experiments and on the people who have the guts to engage in them. At one hospital, managers begin every meeting with a question: "What have you changed lately and why?" In doing so, they spark experimentation, because those who have something to report are recognized. Many hospitals now give innovation awards. These tangible payoffs entice staff to generate experiments and ideas for improvement. The award may be a dinner for two or 10 percent of financial return. One administrator holds "We're off the dime!" parties to celebrate changes.

By informing your staff about innovators in other departments and communicating your admiration and desire to emulate this behavior, you spur your staff to act.

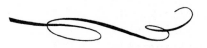

From Busyness to Results

1. Do you overanalyze a problem instead of moving to solve it?   YES   NO
2. Do you spend a lot of time "trying" and much less time "finishing"?   YES   NO
3. Are you more of a problem identifier than a problem solver?   YES   NO
4. Do you make excuses for leaving projects undone?   YES   NO
5. When faced with a difficult situation, do you seek help more often from friends than from experts?   YES   NO
6. Do you become easily discouraged in the face of obstacles?   YES   NO
7. Do you tend to procrastinate on important projects?   YES   NO
8. Do you find that you do not concentrate on projects?   YES   NO
9. Are you known for your intolerance when problems are left unsolved?   YES   NO

10. Do you persist in goal-oriented activity?   YES   NO
11. Do you check on people to whom you have
    delegated work because you feel responsible?   YES   NO
12. When you broach problems with your boss,
    are you prepared to suggest solutions?   YES   NO
13. Do people ever call you tenacious, stubborn,
    persistent, or determined to get what you
    want?   YES   NO
14. Do you lose sleep over problems you have
    not yet been able to solve?   YES   NO
15. Do you work hard because you have to work
    hard if you want results?   YES   NO
16. Do you complete important jobs?   YES   NO

If you answered "yes" to the first eight questions and "no" to the last eight questions, you lean toward keeping busy, working hard, and expending effort. Results are less important to you than the effort you expend. If you answered "no" to the first eight questions and "yes" to the last eight, you judge your value by your results, not by how hard you work.

Managerial Productivity

How common is it in your organization for managers to serve on task forces or standing committees year after year even if these task forces or committees accomplish very little? Because health care organizations of the past could succeed by maintaining business as usual, pressure to produce results at a rapid pace was not the norm. Understandably, managers felt they were doing their jobs when they attended fruitless committee meetings regularly. In our discussions, managers referred to the good old days when you could show up, get your coffee, relax into your chair for a nice long meeting, appear interested, throw some ideas around, and then schedule another meeting to continue the discussion. No results.

This scenario reflects "busyness," working hard whether

or not you obtain results. In contrast, managers with a "results orientation" judge the means by the ends. The means have no intrinsic value. Their value lies in the benefits reaped for the organization.

"Busy" managers may be heard to comment: "We're looking into it further. It's very complex." "Don't worry. I haven't forgotten." "This deserves much more careful study. Let's form a committee." Results-oriented managers are more likely to state: "We're making a decision at the next meeting even if we have to stay all night to do it!" "Maybe it isn't the perfect solution, but it's an improvement and we can't wait forever to act." "Not to decide is to decide."

Managers who value busyness work hard, but not necessarily with efficiency. They see their jobs quantitatively, as hours in the day, number of problems to solve, height of the stack in the in basket, and number of meetings. They make excuses for not finishing tasks. They avoid obstacles and work on less important tasks. They allow themselves to be distracted from what they claim are their priorities. And sometimes, they strive to finish tasks quickly to get them over with, regardless of the quality of the result.

Results-oriented managers, on the other hand, have a clear vision of the results they are working to achieve. They judge their value to the organization by results, not by how hard they work. Turnaround time for decisions and projects tends to be a major concern in their impatience to see results. These managers are decisive, clear in their expectations, and open to finding the best people to help them. Also, they tend to use formal methods to track results on a predetermined schedule. The results-oriented manager is very uncomfortable when things fall through cracks.

Consider how the different types of managers would handle the following cases.

Case 1: Your administrator has asked you to work together with three other managers to improve the hospital's patient transport services. You meet with your group and identify many reasons for the current problems. The results-oriented manager pushes the group to dig deeper into the problems to their root. Then, they attack these with a vengeance by pressing for development of a get-well action plan that can be presented to the administrator. They set an ambitious deadline so that the project does not drag on endlessly.

Case 2: The executive team has asked all department heads to hold a monthly staff meeting to give their staff feedback about the department's performance that month. The "busy" manager focuses on how hard people have been working, difficult situations that arose, and attendance statistics, and, at the end, thanks the staff for giving their all to the organization during such stressful times. The results-oriented manager focuses on satisfaction as reported by customers, problems solved, decisions made, changes instituted, and accomplishments. They also thank staff for contributing to positive results; if the results were negative, they direct people toward improving the results next month.

Case 3: You belong to a committee whose task it is to improve patient education in your hospital. The committee is a diverse group of department managers. You have been meeting many months and have developed no plans. Most members have been arguing over the purpose of the committee. A "busy" manager thinks that committee time does need to be spent clearing the air and that arguing is important until differences are worked out. If this manager becomes impatient with pointless discussion, she or he does little about it because "I'm only one member; I don't have responsibility for this group." Also, this type of manager hesitates to speak up for fear that others might press him or her to take responsibility for the group.

The results-oriented manager knows that the organization cannot afford to have managers waste time in nonproductive meetings. This manager presses for progress by asking "What have we accomplished so far?" "Is this discussion moving us ahead?" "What can we do to move forward to produce a plan?" This manager does not rest until the group has outlined its plan of action, delegated responsibility, and determined deadlines.

The Benefits of Busyness

Managers articulate many benefits of a busyness orientation.

- You feel productive and worth your pay.
- You have a good excuse for saying "no" to almost anything.
- You think you have a great excuse for doing a half-hearted or shoddy job if new demands are made of you; this relieves the pressure.
- You do not have to stretch or challenge yourself or try new things that might be difficult.
- If you held yourself accountable for results, you might have to face failure. It is better to remain in the dark with respect to results.

The hitch is that unless you visibly help the organization achieve results, your value to the organization is in jeopardy. Executives are increasingly less impressed with managers who measure their effectiveness by how hard they work. Executives want managers to produce tangible outcomes that advance the organization's goals.

The Benefits of a Results Orientation

Savvy managers extoll the benefits of a results orientation. And they find the rewards plentiful.

- You can finish projects and experience a feeling of accomplishment.
- You can see change.
- Because you can point to concrete accomplishments, you are more marketable and promotable.
- You gain credibility and respect among staff, among executives, and, increasingly, among peers.
- Because you achieve solutions and move on to other items on your priority list, problems do not accumulate.

- You do not secretly wonder what you could
  have accomplished if you pushed yourself.

Undoubtedly, many organizations will continue to support and sustain "busy" managers. More will not. Whether or not you are forced to be results oriented, examine the costs and benefits of your own style and decide if you are where you want to be.

Strategies That Strengthen Your Results Orientation

A results orientation is a matter of degree. If you want to strengthen yours, here are three, we think unusual and unusually helpful, strategies: (1) Develop a process for monitoring results. (2) Use meeting formats that emphasize results. (3) Push for results one-on-one.

Strategy 1: Develop a process for monitoring results. To hold yourself and your staff accountable for results, you need to monitor performance. Specifically, you need to identify and install indicators that sense the level of performance over time.

We are talking about a scorecard. To focus yourself and your staff on results, keep score on a regular basis and make the scorecard visible to people with the power to improve performance. How is your group doing on key result areas, such as customer satisfaction, timeliness of service delivery, error rates, productivity, and the like.

The measures you use should be related to the results you want. You do not have to be a statistician to measure results efficiently; it takes mostly sweat and common sense, not technical skill. What results do you want to monitor? How can you monitor each? What elements of your service delivery do you want to control? How can you measure them so that you can strengthen results over time?

An enterprising director of medical records translated this desire into action by identifying her department's main customers and their main requirements (key result areas) of her department. Then, for each customer group, she instituted a method for tracking her department's performance in meeting these customer requirements. She began by tracking results related to physician satisfaction, because she pinpointed physicians as her department's priority customer group. Here is the gist of her approach:

Key Customer Requirement 1:
Timely retrieval of patient charts

1. Survey twenty physician users each week. Use short written survey questions:
   - Overall, how quickly did medical records staff retrieve any charts you needed? (scale from 1 to 6)
   - How satisfied were you with the speed of chart retrieval by medical records staff?
2. Have the physicians write *time of request* on the chart request form. The clerk writes the *time delivered* once the chart is retrieved. Each week, the supervisor samples one hundred forms and calculates the number of charts retrieved in a specific time, for example, two minutes, two to five minutes, six to ten minutes.

Key Customer Requirement 2:
Staff courtesy when requesting charts

1. Ask physicians to rate, on a scale of 1-6, how courteous staff were.
2. Count complaints regarding staff discourtesy. Create a log to track these complaints.

To focus her staff on key results in outpatient radiology, another department director developed standards after consulting with patients about their needs and expectations. Like the medical records manager, she measured key result areas, one of which was patient waiting time. When patients who complained of long waits were asked how long a wait they felt was acceptable, most answered twenty minutes. In a staff meeting, the key players decided to set two goals that would be impossible to reach in the short run, but important to work toward to improve patient satisfaction: to see 90 percent of patients within twenty minutes.

The department director arranged with the receptionist to measure the waiting time for all patients on two randomly selected days per week for twenty-one weeks. At the end of each week, she summarized the results and plotted the data on a trend chart (Figure 9) designed to show the discrepancy between her department's performance and target performance. Such charts make the results tangible. One picture is worth a thousand words.

Figure 9. Waiting-Time Trend Chart.

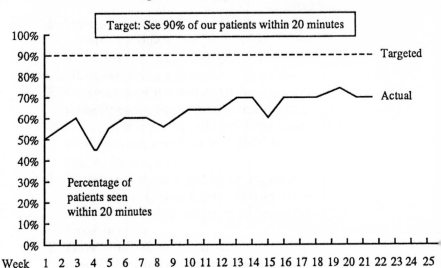

Source: Albert Einstein Healthcare Foundation, from "Service Management Essentials," Module 4 of the Service Quality Improvement Process. © 1989.

When people receive feedback about their performance, they initiate corrective action almost as a reflex. If, while driving along a road, your car hits the curb, you quickly turn the wheel to get back on course. Similarly do workers take corrective action when they receive constructive feedback, often without formal problem solving.

Skeptical? Note this relevant and real example: One enormous health maintenance organization (HMO) with physician shareholders had received more than enough complaints about the behavior of some of their physicians toward patients. The HMO provided education in interpersonal skills for the physicians, but to no avail. Then they decided to institute a simple feedback system that would provide each physician with customer satisfaction information relevant to him or her. The HMO distributed short survey forms to all patients after their appointments. The physicians were given feedback and also were told how they ranked among their peers. As a result, the physicians improved their behavior. The feedback forced the physicians to focus on their behavior *and* held them accountable. They were confronted with the consequences of their actions.

Feedback can be just as powerful for you and your staff. You cannot know if you are winning if you do not keep score!

Strategy 2: Use meeting formats that emphasize results. Three meeting formats can be used to encourage a results orientation: (1) results review meeting, (2) stand-up meeting, and (3) marathon meeting.

You have instituted a process for monitoring results and have displayed those results in a trend chart. Now you must present these results to your staff and engage them in drawing conclusions and planning appropriate action in a results review meeting.

Distribute the most recent trend chart for each key result area monitored. Ask your staff to peruse it and share their reactions to these results. If the results are positive, ask them what worked well to produce the positive results. If the results exceed previously set performance targets, celebrate.

If performance falls short of expectations, discuss the circumstances and root causes. Now, engage your staff in revising your performance target for the next measurement period, making sure this revised target is both ambitious and achievable. Finally, generate and commit to a plan for the actions or changes needed to reach the new targets.

Some 60 percent of a manager's time is consumed in

meetings. When you ask managers how well this time is spent, the typical response is laughter. Many managers agree that they "relax" into meetings: "You sink into the chair, sip your coffee, and unwind a bit, even though the task at hand might be quite important." To prevent this "settling in" syndrome, consider a stand-up meeting. Research shows that people make decisions much more quickly when standing rather than sitting, and the quality of the decisions does not differ. Apparently, one's circulation is enhanced in the standing position. Generally, a standing person is more alert, permitting enhanced concentration on the subject at hand.

How does a stand-up meeting work? Picture a huddle. You remove the chairs from the room and tell people that you believe efficiency will be enhanced and precious time will be conserved if they stand during the meeting. A typical stand-up meeting lasts ten minutes, whereas a traditional meeting with the same agenda averages an hour. People tend not to repeat themselves or talk for the sake of hearing themselves talk if they are standing. Perhaps they are motivated to make the necessary decisions so they can find a seat!

Marathon meetings are at the other extreme. Imagine that your meeting goal takes longer to achieve than the time scheduled for the meeting. So you convene more meetings in an attempt to reach a conclusion. It seems highly inefficient, because each meeting begins with a review of previous meetings. To stop this endless cycle, schedule a marathon meeting. Get the group to agree to lock themselves in a room (with meals delivered) until you can all reach a decision. To avoid fatigue and possibly an "all-nighter," staff will demonstrate unexpected, sometimes shocking levels of efficiency, attention, and decisiveness. Marathons break the cycle of perfunctory meetings and the accompanying busyness that rarely produces resource-efficient results.

The point is that as manager, you can structure meetings that propel you and your staff toward a results orientation. And you will have more results to show for your efforts.

Strategy 3: Push for results one-on-one. Your language has the power to influence others' priorities and actions. Use these key questions to focus individuals on results. The more often you ask the questions, the better.

- Since I saw you last, what results have you improved? What results concern you?
- Are you not satisfied with the result? What do you plan to do about it?
- Why are you doing this? To make what happen?
- What are you trying to achieve?
- What is your point in describing this situation?
- When can I expect the finished product?
- What have you improved lately?

The determination to achieve results is needed today. And it takes hard work, without a doubt.

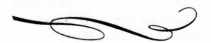

9

From Turf Protection to Teamwork Across Lines

1. Do you mind your own business, even when activity or inactivity in another department is obviously interfering with your staff's effectiveness?   YES   NO

2. Do you resent it when other managers tell you something negative about your department?   YES   NO

3. Do you hesitate to ask for help from other managers because you are afraid they will see you as incompetent?   YES   NO

4. When you have a problem in your department, do you think you should be able to solve it on your own, without involving other people?   YES   NO

5. Have you resigned yourself to the difficulties involved in interdepartmental problem solving to the point where you avoid it as much as possible?   YES   NO

6. Do you avoid asking other managers for help with problems and projects unless they are key actors in the problem or project?   YES   NO

7. Are you cynical about the possibility of solving problems that cut across departmental lines because other people will not do their share of the work?   YES   NO
8. Do you find yourself feeling defensive when others in the organization complain about your practices or people?   YES   NO
9. Do other managers avoid asking you for help?   YES   NO
10. Would other managers in the organization characterize you as territorial?   YES   NO

Managers who answer "Yes" to most of the preceding items are inclined to devote their time and energy to advancing their own department and protecting their turf rather than contributing to the overall performance of the organization through teamwork.

Crossing Lines

Once upon a time, managers could mind their own business without dire consequences. Hospitals were not threatened by competitive forces or resource constraints, so status quo management was adequate to the task. Problems beyond the scope of one manager were ignored. Crossing lines was simply not worth the aggravation. Not only that! In the large bureaucracies, managers worked hard to build strong group identity among their own staff, so that the staff would not feel insignificant.

Consider the following scenario: For years, Hospital XYZ has been plagued by the unavailability of wheelchairs in several key locations, especially the front lobby and the emergency room. In an initial investigation, it was found that the hospital had a very high ratio of wheelchairs to patients and that these wheelchairs were in good repair. At least seven different departments were acutely affected and frustrated by this shortage. Yet, the problem had become legendary, and no substantial attempts to solve it had been made in years.

The department director in charge of transportation services threw his hands in the air with frustration, blaming the nurses in the emergency room for hoarding wheelchairs behind locked doors where the right people could not get them when needed. When the director of the emergency room heard this accusation, she was shocked and angry, because the emergency room had never been able to count on transportation services to provide wheelchairs in a timely or reliable fashion. Also, she proceeded to point out that the volunteers leave the wheelchairs on the floors "wherever the patient gets out." The director of volunteers defended her people and pointed out that the nurses on the floors push the chairs aside where no one can find them. Other department managers blamed the problem on administrators "who seem to focus on everything but what's important." And on and on.

When asked to share his or her diagnosis of the problem, each key player in the wheelchair shortage blamed another for the problem and expressed extreme frustration about his or her powerlessness.

Such problems have extreme consequences for the daily routine. Service to patients is impeded, and staff are frustrated as they chase around the hospital to find wheelchairs. Yet, the problem continues. Why? Because every manager involved feels powerless to institute solutions. They see themselves as owning only a small piece of the problem. For instance, if ten departments are involved in such a problem, each manager feels ownership of, at most, 10 percent of the problem. To them, that is nothing, so they do not feel they have to solve it. Or, they may be reluctant to work with other managers on the problem, because they believe these other managers do not want to be bothered and will blame them for the problem. So the problem persists and time and energy continue to be wasted.

So many important problems are interdepartmental, especially systems problems that involve the flow of patients, paperwork, and communication. These problems are extremely difficult to solve, not because they are unsolvable, but because managers think and act as turf protectors rather than team players. Turf protectors create enormous divisions between departments that prevent staff from working together to solve problems and seize opportunities.

Today teamwork, not turf protection, is a business necessity. The problems that have persisted because of the lack of teamwork are simply too costly for the organization to tolerate. Our organizations must become "seamless" and only managers can make that happen.

Turf-protecting managers do not trust other managers. They compete with them for resources without regard for the good of the entire organization. They screen news, information, requests, and decisions from the perspective of how it will affect their department and their people.

Turf protectors blame people from other departments for problems, even for those problems in which they are involved. They avoid making waves or pressing for changes that involve others.

Team players, on the other hand, devote energy and time to building relationships between departments to achieve the mutual support needed to solve problems and institute changes. They recognize and care about the effects of their practices, problems, and decisions on other departments, other people, and the entire organization.

Administrators commonly associate the following words and phrases with turf-protecting managers: mine, selfish, isolated, minds own business, plays it safe, hiding, hoarding, competitive, suspicious, possessive, tunnel vision, defensive, blaming, not a team player. Words and phrases they associate with team players are supportive, risk taker, cooperative, interdependent, open to compromise, reasonable, helpful, and team player. The value judgments are clear.

Consider the differences between turf protectors and team players in response to two situations.

Case 1: A physician complains to you about a problem he is having with another department. You ask the physician if he has discussed the problem with that department's director. The physician answers, "He doesn't like me. There is no point in speaking up." The turf-protecting manager makes sure the physician was not complaining about her department, and once reassured of this, she thanks her lucky stars. Her involvement ends there. The team player manager encourages the physician to speak to the appropriate department director, expressing confidence in her colleague's likely responsiveness. Also, she probably initiates a conversation with the other manager in the spirit of helpfulness and support, sharing the incident with him and expressing her expectation that he would welcome this feedback.

Case 2: Your organization wants to institute a satisfaction guarantee program that would provide patients with a hotline number they could call to obtain an immediate response to problems. No money is available for additional staff. Your department already manages a twenty-four-hour line for doctors who want an immediate response. Your staff could probably handle patient calls as well. The turf protector does not admit that his staff can handle the extra work. He claims to need more staff or resources to handle patient calls. Why take on more work without getting anything for it?

The team player discusses the additional work with staff and carefully investigates the department's capacity to do it. If they believe they can handle the calls, the manager suggests they conduct a trial during which they will track call volume and integrate the service into their department without new resources.

The Costs and Benefits of Turf Protection Versus Teamwork

No doubt, turf protection has reaped tremendous benefits, as such managers strongly resist changing their style:

- You feel more successful when you focus only on forces immediately within your control, on your turf. If you deal only with your own area's needs, you have a whole lot less to do than you would if you cared about things beyond your turf. And you can do things your own way; you don't have to work out problems or decisions with other managers.

- You have a piece of turf to call your own in an otherwise large, complex organization. You're a big fish in a little pond, instead of a little fish in a big pond. Staff see you as their protectors, advocates, and allies. They appreciate you. And since you're with them much more than you're with anyone else, that makes the work more comfortable.

- It's easier to blame other departments for your problems than to solve them yourself.

- You don't have to challenge the age-old taboo in your organization against crossing turf lines; if you did challenge it, you would get flack from peers.

Although these benefits are real, the costs of turf protection, and the benefits of teamwork, are on the rise.

Turf protectors are not viewed as team players, and today team players are sought and valued by the powers that be. If you are turf oriented, you inevitably harbor anxiety-provoking feelings of competitiveness, isolation, and defensiveness. You cannot count on feedback or support from peers in tough situations, because those peers expect you to be defensive. You have a very hard time solving problems or getting things done, because so many of the important problems and projects require interdepartmental action. And, you probably feel alone, because your peers steer clear of your area.

Teamworking managers feel the support of peers. They accomplish more because they can approach and rely on other departments for help. They can also take greater risks because, by taking these risks with others, they enjoy "safety in numbers" and achieve solutions that would otherwise be impossible. They also feel more committed to and more confident in the organization.

Turf-to-Team Continuum

Crossing turf boundaries to work as a team is a matter of degree and it does not happen overnight. If you and your colleagues want to be team players, consider the turf-to-team continuum, which illustrates the steps involved.

Turf-to-Team Continuum

Turf
1 Information sharing
2 Sense making
3 Mutual consulting
4 Interdepartmental problem solving and planning
5 Whole group decision making and implementation
▼ 6 Group activism and advocacy

Team

At point 1, information sharing, managers exchange facts and perceptions. The individual must decide whether to use what has been learned to plan actions. Managers are, at the least, more informed.

At point 2, sense making, managers discuss the information they have shared and together derive conclusions and implications. There is no pressure to reach a consensus or make decisions. It is up to the individual to use the conclusions or implications.

At point 3, mutual consultation, managers help each other with problems or projects facing one of them. It is up to the individual to act on the substance of the consultation.

At point 4, interdepartmental problem solving and planning, all managers affected by a problem or project work together on it; they develop and debug the plan and then divide responsibility for its implementation.

At point 5, whole group decision making and implementation, managers work on problems, make group decisions, divide responsibility for implementation, and commit themselves to follow through.

At point 6, group activism and advocacy, managers work on a problem, develop a position as a group, and act together for its adoption, even if risk and confrontation of the powers-that-be are necessary.

To move along this continuum, talk with colleagues about where you are, where you want to be, and how you want to get there step by step.

Strategies That Move You from Turf to Team

Although there are myriad ways to institutionalize activity along the continuum, in Table 1 you will find a meeting format that triggers success at each point. The strategies summarized in Table 1 are explained in greater detail in the text.

Strategy 1: Sharing/problems/plans. The sharing/problems/plans meeting format encourages the widespread, efficient sharing of information among managers. "Sharing/problems/plans" (SPP) works like this. Before a meeting begins, managers consider any bits of sharing, problems, or plans they want to discuss with other managers. If so, they write their initials on an "agenda board" (Exhibit 6) to reserve time during the relevant section of the meeting for their contribution.

Sharing is first on the agenda. Those who sign up for this portion of the meeting talk about an experience or report a new discovery, an accomplishment, an idea, or a feeling. The subject may be related to work or personal. "Sharing" time gives the group a chance to focus on its members as people, not simply workers, as these excerpts from a meeting illustrate:

- Our department just conducted a terrific course on marketing. We've been getting calls from people about it and are really excited. Here's a quick description of what we did.

- I went to a conference in New York last week and got some great ideas about some new ways to handle walk-in appointments.

- My wife was just promoted to president of her bank.

Table 1. Turf-to-Team Strategies in a Nutshell.

Point on Continuum	Strategy	Nutshell Summary
Information sharing	Sharing/problems/ plans	Managers share information about their activities, problems, and plans.
Sense making	Peer discussion forums	Managers engage in processing information together; ideal after meetings with or communications from senior management.
Mutual consultation	Mutual consultation	Every manager has a chance to solicit the advice and perspective of peers on a problem he or she faces.
Interdepartmental problem solving and planning	Liaison teams	Managers engage in working together on problems that cut across departmental lines.
Whole group decision making and implementation	Greenhouse meetings	Managers have opportunities to tackle problems and design innovations that they have the power to implement using their combined resources.
Group activism and advocacy	"Making our case" groups	Managers work together to make decisions about what they want to make happen that requires senior management approval and/or investment, and to build a powerful case for it that they will all support.

Exhibit 6. Agenda Board

Sharing	Problems	Plans
R.M. A.P.	S.C.	L.L. B.R. L.D. G.S.

People can also sign up to discuss a problem related to work, other staff members, or customers. The problem section of the meeting is intended to identify, not solve, problems. The manager who identifies the problem might, however, ask for volunteers to help at a later meeting or over lunch.

People can also present plans to the group. These plans might be for events in their department that they want to publicize, proposals they want to make, or projects that require the involvement of other managers.

At each meeting, one manager volunteers to be navigator, keeping the meeting on course. SPP meetings can be held weekly, biweekly, or monthly. They are flexible and can be adapted to the time constraints and style of an individual group to produce productive meetings that induce communication.

SPP meetings work best in groups smaller than twenty. With large groups, ask people to sign the agenda board *before* the meeting. Then, a subcommittee can prioritize the agenda and postpone some items.

Strategy 2: Peer discussion forums. Peer discussion forums provide an opportunity for managers to process information together and share conclusions and perceptions regarding its meaning and implications.

Ideally, such forums are held immediately after meetings at which senior management conveys dense information. The interested managers convene, without executives present, to share their reactions. Executives who feel threatened by this should be reminded that they have asked repeatedly for less passivity on the part of managers when faced with information.

In the peer discussion forum, share personal impressions first: What information surprised you? Why? What disturbed you? Why? What were you glad to hear? Why? Then, share conclusions: What does this mean to the organization? Our customers? Your department? Your staff? You?

Single-topic peer discussion forums are also powerful. Reserve a room once a week for a brown-bag lunch that interested managers attend voluntarily. Topics can be suggested ahead of time, or a committee can develop an agenda each month. Use the "what/so what/now what" format:

- What is the issue?
- So what? Why is it worth our attention? What does it mean to us?
- Now what? Given what it means to us, what should we do about it? What are possible responses?

Strategy 3: Mutual consultation. The following simple format for mutual consultation gives managers a chance to solicit help on problems or projects they are facing. Start by dividing your group into threes. Then, twenty minutes is devoted to each member of the trio.

1. One manager describes the problem/project. The others ask clarifying questions.
2. To ensure that the problem is understood, the other members restate it in their own words. One definition of the problem is chosen by the original speaker.
3. Solutions are brainstormed.
4. The manager who presented the problem selects one or

two suggestions to explore further. He or she is expected to report progress to the group at the next meeting.
5.   This process is repeated for the remaining two managers.

Strategy 4: Liaison teams. Liaison teams help managers to build the necessary bridges between their departments that facilitate communication. This vehicle operationalizes activity at the fourth point on the continuum, interdepartmental problem solving and planning.

Liaison teams involve only *two* departments. One hospital set up eighteen such teams, including nursing–pharmacy, utilization review–social services, nursing–laboratories, admissions–nursing, plant operations–nursing, and unit management–physician relations.

The team should comprise at least one department manager (director or assistant director), supervisors, and staff. Typically, a team is composed of four to eight people, with equal representation of the two departments.

Because only two departments are involved, their managers develop a partnership in approaching problems that would otherwise disappear in the gulf that separates them.

Strategy 5: Greenhouse meetings. Greenhouse meetings trigger solutions and innovations that can be implemented only with the combined resources of all the managers involved. The point here is to talk about possibilities, nurture ideas, design initiatives, and make them happen. If senior management is urging you to "run with the ball at your level," you can generate an extensive and even surprising array of solutions and innovations in a freewheeling greenhouse meeting:

- Decide what you want to do.
- Develop an airtight plan, including measures to overcome anticipated obstacles.
- Check with one another about whether "permission" is needed from superiors or whether this plan is within the power and resources of the managers.

- Divide responsibilities and contract with one another to fulfill them.
- Decide who will serve as the clearinghouse for progress and problems—a project coordinator.
- Schedule the next meeting.
- Decide who will "inform" senior management about what is happening and report back to the group the nature of this communication.

Strategy 6: "Making our case" groups. "Making our case" groups provide managers with the tools needed to become "of one mind" on a goal that involves senior management approval. Managers are able to make their case.

The following steps (adapted from the Blueprint for Making Your Case described in Chapter Six) constitute an excellent format for a support group discussion, in preparation for a group advocacy role:

1. Clarify your goals.
2. Identify your reasons—for customers, your department, the organization, and others.
3. Identify the key people or groups whose support you need.
4. Anticipate the reasons they might resist and plan to address these. Determine in great detail the costs and risks involved. Show that you have thought through everything carefully and are not proceeding blindly.
5. Spell out in great detail all possible benefits for you, your staff, your department, the administration, your boss in particular, the organization, and your organization's customers. Obtain or project numbers to document these benefits. When possible, compare future benefits with past statistics.
6. Now put it all together. Articulate your case so that your superiors are convinced they cannot *live* without your idea.
7. Remain confident and assertive. Expect the people you address to realize you are making sense and support the proposal. If they do not support it, act surprised. Persist.

If you still get a "no" but you remain convinced that the organization is making a big mistake, work with your peer group to revise your approach, trying a different angle.

The Basic Ingredients to Teamwork: Openness and Trust

To make any of these strategies work, you need to trust one another. Defensiveness and distrust block constructive teamwork.

Support is manifested not by unconditional approval, but by honest and direct feedback, constructive conflict, and communication. You are in a very tough spot if you are caught between unloving critics and uncritical admirers. Sure, you need reassurance, but you also need advisors, colleagues who will guide you with care and candor through the mine fields.

To operate effectively as a team player, resist acting defensively in response to honest and direct feedback from peers. If you act like all is rosy when it really is not, you isolate yourself from help and support. If you will not tolerate criticism and the free expression of problems, possibilities, ideas, and reactions, teamwork is no more than rhetoric to you.

Some managers claim that tough interdepartmental problems remain unsolved because managers do not trust one another to implement even brilliant solutions. Returning to the wheelchair shortage, after agreement is reached on a system for the timely return of wheelchairs, some managers may choose not to trust their colleagues to enforce the solution and hoard wheelchairs "just in case." The solution thus becomes ineffective quickly. Once one person hoards, the system breaks down and others hoard too. Managers who decide to work as a team must face the issue of trust and, perhaps, build in checks and balances that permit more experimentation.

Managers at one hospital in Virginia develop "responsibility contracts" between peers. If a manager thinks another manager is not holding up his or her end of the agreement, that manager initiates a grievance process with the peer council. The peer council, established at the time responsibilities are negotiated, investigates the situation and follows through to ensure that the responsibilities are fulfilled. The distrust among managers is reduced because there now exists a system that promotes trust by enforcing accountability.

To change from a turf protector to a team player, you must reexamine and modify the long-held patterns of thought and action previously supported by organizations. You must build the bridges that lead to new power and new opportunities.

From "We-They" Thinking to Organizational Perspective

1. Do you accept responsibility for helping employees understand difficult administrative decisions so that they retain their faith in the organization and senior management? YES NO
2. Do you take the initiative to obtain information from senior management when you feel uninformed, instead of resenting being in the dark? YES NO
3. Do you ask your staff for suggestions and ideas about how the organization, not only your department, can be strengthened? YES NO
4. Do you feel a strong identity with the organization? YES NO
5. Do you take active steps to help your staff respect the functions and plight of employees in other departments, to decrease interdepartmental divisiveness? YES NO
6. Do you keep information about the organization's status from employees for fear it will dampen their morale? YES NO

7. Do you openly criticize administrative decisions with your staff?   YES   NO
8. Do you find yourself resenting decisions that
   affect your own staff negatively, even if you
   know these decisions are wise for the organization?   YES   NO
9. Do you openly discuss with your staff nega-
   tive perceptions you have of other departments?   YES   NO
10. Do you find yourself supporting or ignoring
    negative comments made by your staff about
    other departments?   YES   NO

"Yes" answers to the first five questions indicate a tendency toward organizational perspective, whereas "yes"
answers to the last five questions indicate a tendency toward
"we-they" thinking.

As times get tougher and work gets harder, executives
need more from the work force. They need people who will
roll with the punches, do more with less, and take on new
responsibilities in a spirit of teamwork to help the organization survive and thrive. This is a very tall order for employees
who are overstressed, insecure about their jobs, and pessimistic about their future.

To secure the cooperation of employees, executives
must rely on managers to nurture employee loyalty to the
organization. Executives look to managers to be supportive
spokespersons who convey messages to the work force and
report back reactions, concerns, questions, and problems so
that senior management can stay in touch.

Managers have always had to walk this tightrope
between senior management and staff. Managers must cater
to two constituencies, wear two hats. This role has been made
more difficult because of tough new environmental conditions
and constraints. Executives are forced to make tough decisions that have implications painful to many employees.

Managers feel caught in the middle. They want the best
for their employees, on the one hand, and they want to sup-

port executive decisions for the sake of the organization on the other. Walking this tightrope becomes especially difficult when managers disagree with the actions and priorities of superiors.

So, what does the effective manager do? Do you let your true feelings show or do you mask them? What is best for your staff, the organization, and your own integrity is not obvious.

What is clear is that health care organizations need managers who can ride the rapids while keeping staff confident in the organization. For many managers, this requires a shift from "we-they" thinking to a broader organizational perspective and visible loyalty.

"We-They" Managers

"We-they" managers are concerned largely with their department's best interests, not those of the organization. They see their role as protecting their resources, even if other departments are in greater need of these resources. They are concerned with the big picture only as it affects their people. They disagree publicly with senior management. They resent decisions that adversely affect their department, even if these decisions make excellent sense for the organization and its customers. In short, they feel no responsibility for making senior management look good or for building their staff's confidence in the organization and its future.

"We-they" managers are strong advocates for their staffs. Their staffs are not their primary loyalty, but their only loyalty.

Managers with an Organizational Perspective

Managers who act on organizational perspective operate very differently from "we-they" managers. In the face of unwelcome news, they seek the facts because they believe employees deserve substantive information. They ask the tough questions so they can learn the truth and come up with the right answers. They accept responsibility for securing employee acceptance of difficult decisions.

Organizational thinkers foster interdepartmental communication on the grounds that the organization, its customers, and its staff all benefit from bridges, not walls. They even bring discordant parties together to foster unity. And they actively help employees understand the jobs, responsibilities, frustrations, accomplishments, and needs of other employees throughout the organization.

Consider the difference in approach between "we-they" managers and organizational thinkers in four familiar case situations.

Case 1: You and other managers have been told that certain employee benefits will be cut across the board. The rationale given is that the hospital needs to save several million dollars this fiscal year. Department budgets had already been cut. You are asked to communicate this news to your staff. Managers are often asked to communicate such news to employees. When the organization's financial problems begin to affect salaries and benefits, it is not easy for managers to keep the faith. Employees feel they are disadvantaged enough from the stress they endure.

Some "we-they" managers convey openly to their staff their own feelings of frustration and resentment toward the executive team whom they paint as misguided or even ogreish. Such behavior triggers destructive feelings. Other "we-they" managers feel so uncomfortable communicating bad news that they avoid it and wait until staff find out via memos or the grapevine.

Managers with an organizational perspective seek to understand and become comfortable with the decision. Discovering the underlying reasons helps the manager resolve his or her own mixed feelings before talking with employees. Then, when they talk with employees, they have all the facts and, therefore, more credibility. When these managers do not receive the full story up front, they press senior management for more facts and their implications.

Case 2: You have just been informed that your depart-

ment will be merged with two other departments. You will share space and support staff and also report to one boss. You must explain this to your people. You are disturbed about the decision and you know your people will be too. The most difficult aspect of this problem is probably the manager's own feelings about the changes. Clearly, employees take cues and direction from their managers. The "we-they" manager makes the announcement and lets the chips fall where they may.

Organizational thinkers come to terms with the decision, work out its implications with the other departments involved, and resolve their own negativity before telling their employees. They communicate honestly with their employees about their initial feelings and how they worked them through to a point where, now, they embrace the plan and will do all they can to make it work.

Case 3: Your hospital is launching a series of awareness-raising, skill-building programs designed to strengthen the respect, compassion, and courtesy all employees extend toward patients and their loved ones. According to the scuttlebutt, staff nurses feel that other employees (housekeeping, linen, pharmacy, and other support departments) need these programs but not them. "We-they" nurse managers quickly agree with their staff. They resist scheduling their staff to attend until forced to do so by senior management. Others may schedule nurses to attend but maintain that the nurses do not need these programs because they are so obviously superior to support personnel with respect to "caring behavior."

Nurse managers with an organizational perspective work hard to embrace the purpose and approach of the strategy being undertaken. Instead of defending nurses as separate and apart from other employees in their need for this refresher, they insist that *all* employees can benefit and actively voice their support of the programs.

Case 4: Your hospital merged with two other hospitals two years ago. In that time your hospital has done very well financially. The other two hospitals have not been as successful. Your people feel they are being dragged down by the other hospitals and resent it. The "we-they" manager agrees and voices resentment freely with staff, thereby giving them permission to continue resisting reality. Such managers would also fight efforts by the executive team to build a corporate identity and to foster collaboration across lines.

Managers loyal to the organization would, on the other hand, take substantial time to explain the reasons for the merger; they would emphasize the potential to build a stronger organization better equipped to survive in the current environment and better able to meet the community's health needs. If these managers were upset by the merger, they would admit their concerns calmly and proceed to embrace a realistic positive outlook, showing staff that they have come to terms with the merger and will do all they can to make it work. They would urge staff to do their best to give the merger a chance, to support people from the other hospitals, and to cooperate with them.

In situations such as those just described, managers need to help employees broaden their perspective. In some instances, the manager must share more information tactfully or obtain the information that is lacking. Employees must learn to see things from someone else's point of view. Different groups must overcome differences and achieve an understanding and compromise.

In all of these situations, the manager risks disapproval and rejection. These situations tend to be threatening and uncomfortable. But, executives seek and support managers who take the initiative, obtain the necessary information, stick their necks out, and boldly support the organization. The degree of stability and confidence possible today depends on the management team's ability to present a united front.

Costs and Benefits of "We-They" Versus Organizational Perspective

"We-they" management has its benefits. These managers do not risk disapproval by their staff because they focus exclusively on their staff's needs. They always have someone to blame for things they do not like and changes that are difficult. They do not expend effort viewing events from a perspective broader than their own tunnel vision. "We-they" managers are not accused of brownnosing. And, perhaps most important, the "we-they" manager fosters strong group identity within the department by painting outsiders as enemies.

Although these benefits are compelling, the countervailing costs of "we-they" management are even more compelling. In today's environment, our organizations require teamwork and loyalty to meet the challenges facing them. "We-they" managers must know, deep down, that encouraging divisiveness hurts the organization, because it consumes precious energy with infighting and slows progress. Also, staff are demoralized when they watch change rather than be a part of it. More managers now realize that although "we-they" management gains approval from staff, approval is not the same as respect. Managers who reflect and breed organizational thinking and loyalty are valued as team players.

Managers who have overcome "we-they" thinking to embrace organizational perspective report these benefits:

- I know I'm really doing the job I was hired to do and that I'm ultimately making life easier for my staff and my boss.
- I feel more positive and so do my staff, probably because there just isn't as much backbiting and finger pointing. And, you know that when people are backbiting and finger pointing, they are not working or taking responsibility for their part in problems.
- I feel much more respected by my colleagues and the administration than I used to. Or maybe I'm just feeling better about my role— more honest really.
- You can feel proud knowing that you are contributing to a healthy, productive organization.
- I'm impressed by how much you can do when you see other people as allies instead of as enemies.

"We-they" management is hazardous to morale and productivity.

Strategies That Foster an Organizational Perspective

To discourage "we-they" thinking and foster identification with and loyalty to the overall organization, keep your staff informed not only about your department but also about the organization. It is inevitable that you will, as managers, have to convey bad news; you need to do so while maintaining your staff's confidence in the organization. And, you need to help staff widen their perspective. Use the following strategies to help you accomplish these goals: (1) Share the big picture. (2) Communicate in a manner that keeps the faith. (3) Help your staff walk in others' shoes.

Strategy 1: Share the big picture. Your staff need and deserve substantial, truthful, and frequent information about the organization to feel committed to it. We learned this years ago when we worked with hospital employees to implement long-range service excellence strategies. In focus groups, employees told us how they would feel if the hospital instituted an explicit service strategy. We asked them what could be done to win their commitment and involvement. One woman from housekeeping piped up, "If you want my commitment, you'd better get management to tell the truth about why we're doing this. They can't expect me to get on any bandwagon unless they tell me the truth about it—the whole truth. I guess this administration thinks we're too dumb to understand the big picture. Well, if that's true, then they can't expect my commitment!"

Other members of the group echoed her sentiments. Employees will not be loyal to the organization unless they think "organization," not "department." Share with them the challenges faced by the organization and what is being done to meet those challenges. Explain how they can contribute to the success of the organization. If you shelter employees from the truth, you are the root cause of their tunnel vision.

Two techniques work very well to communicate the big picture: "what's new?" updates and "ask me" meetings.

A "what's new" update is like a state-of-the-union address. It is a straightforward presentation that covers the following questions:

- What challenges has our organization faced lately, for example, industry trends, reimbursement constraints, image problems, increasing public scrutiny, competition, alternative providers, staffing shortages, morale problems?
- How is our organization responding to each challenge, for example, number of admissions, patient satisfaction, ability to attract talented physicians, vacancy rates, financial viability in atmosphere of reimbursement and resource constraints?
- What are we doing to succeed? What are our success strategies, for example, physician recruitment campaigns, market research, new services, centers of excellence, improvement in service quality, customer feedback systems?
- Where does our department fit? What can we do to help the organization address the challenges we face, for example, do a quality job, initiate improvements, extend excellent service to every customer, cross departmental lines to solve problems?

This information is very important to employees. Without it, sympathy with leaders' decisions and loyalty to the organization cannot be expected.

In some organizations, senior management addresses these questions in around-the-clock sessions for all employees. If these are not conducted in your organization, consider joining together with other managers to urge senior management to provide them. Or, get the information you need and provide them yourself.

"Ask me" meetings provide excellent interim reinforcement of "what's new?" updates. "Ask me" meetings are question-and-answer sessions in which you encourage staff to do the asking. You can answer or you can invite your superior to help. Sparking direct interaction between your superior and your staff humanizes the "they" group; employees learn that administrators are people too, and your superior listens to employee concerns directly.

In our experience, these meetings work best if you are up-front about the purpose. Consider one manager's explanation:

> I feel very committed to this organization. I know where we're heading and I want to do my part to help. I want you [my staff] to feel committed too. This "ask me" meeting is a chance for you to ask questions, so you'll have a good grasp of what's happening with our organization and know your important role and how you can help.
>
> Ask me anything. If I don't know the answer, I'll find it out. If I feel uncomfortable answering your question for some reason, I'll admit it and explain why I feel uncomfortable. For any question I need time to look into, I'll write up the answer for you by next week.
>
> As I see it, this organization needs all of us to keep it thriving. And I know, for you to feel committed and loyal—and that's what I want you to feel—you need and deserve to know what's happening around here. So, shoot! Ask me anything.

Strategy 2: Communicate in a manner that keeps the faith. When you have to justify to staff the reasons for organizational change, *how* you communicate—your style and language—powerfully influences staff feelings, either fueling "we-they" thinking or nurturing organizational perspective.

Consider how you communicate unpopular decisions or bad news, for example, no raise, job freeze, unfillable vacancies, an increase in patient complaints, notice of a move, accreditation problems, and financial problems. As you know, it is difficult to relay such information, especially when you have not been involved in the decision.

In the delicate role of messenger, you need to communicate the news in the best light possible.

To help people make the best of bad news, we offer the following suggestions:

- Keep your perspective. Unpopular decisions and occasional setbacks are a normal part of organizational life.
- Be realistic and truthful about what people can expect. If you are, staff may be unhappy or angry, but they will be less likely to blow up.
- Tell your employees before they hear the news from others. Word travels fast, and people resent hearing news from peers that you should have communicated to them first.
- Choose your method carefully. Even though you might feel more comfortable sending a memo, you show much more concern when you talk face-to-face.
- Get right to the point. Discussing other business or building spirit by praising employees first only increases tension.
- Show confidence in other managers and the executive team. If you say "I don't know why they did this" or "Guess what they're making us do now?" you only encourage resentment.
- Encourage employees to react to the news. This lessens their need to vent in less constructive ways when they are beyond earshot.
- Listen with empathy. Acknowledge strong feelings and group sentiment without taking sides.
- Show that you are confident, forward looking, and in control. Tell employees your plans for helping the department deal with the consequences of the news constructively.

Also, consider confirming and explaining difficult decisions in writing, so that everyone has the same story. One manager summarized and confirmed a difficult layoff decision in a memo (Exhibit 7). She wanted her staff to understand it and survive it with no more than inevitable pain. Note the language in the memo.

Exhibit 7. Memo Confirming Oral Communication of Bad News.

To: Staff
From: Rita
Subject: Downsizing of Our Department

In the face of a dramatic budget cut and after exploring a variety of alternatives, I have made a series of decisions that I believe are necessary to secure our department's future. Painfully, I must tell you that these involve elimination of several positions and loss of valued, beloved, and dedicated members of our team.
The following positions are being eliminated:

- The position of secretary held by Cindy
- The position of supervisor held by Margaret
- The position of clerk held by Ralph

Why the Need to Reduce Staff?
Elimination of these positions has nothing to do with job performance. The people involved have shown exemplary performance— hard work, excellent customer service, tremendous talent in their areas of expertise, and teamwork.
The elimination of positions at this time is necessary because of the enormous deficit our hospital faces unless it reduces expenses by millions of dollars. This huge deficit is a result of government reimbursement rule changes for the hospital industry as a whole and drastic cuts in state subsidies to teaching hospitals for medical education. At our hospital, entire patient care programs are being eliminated as a result.
In this atmosphere, in good conscience, our executive team decided that we had to share in the burden of cost reductions by reducing the size of our department's budget. And, in our case, since we have already cut nonstaff expenses to the bone, this means eliminating positions.

In Summary
The turbulence of the health care marketplace is having its impact on us. We are not exempt from the cutbacks and upheaval top-notch hospitals have been experiencing. I can only hope that the turbulence and upheaval this means for people personally will turn into opportunities for growth, productive work, and personal fulfillment.
These are painful times for us. We will miss Cindy, Margaret, and Ralph personally and professionally. I know I can count on you to do all you can to be supportive of one another during these times. Please do not hesitate to ask questions, make suggestions, or ask for any help you might want during this painful transition.
This afternoon, at 2 P.M., I will be holding a meeting in our conference room to address any questions you might have about these decisions and plans and to promote discussion among us.

Another critical opportunity you have to build or erode organizational perspective revolves around your behavior surrounding organizational change efforts. If your organization has launched or is planning to launch product-line management, a far-reaching new management information system, a service excellence strategy, a total quality improvement effort, new interdepartmental systems, or the like, you are called upon to support these efforts with wholehearted commitment. If you do, you engender commitment and feelings of investment among your staff.

How you communicate your own attitude toward these efforts at change is pivotal to employee involvement. If you resist change and let it show, you breed resistance among your staff and colleagues.

Recently, many health care organizations have instituted strategies to achieve service excellence with the purpose of heightening customer satisfaction. Typically, the administrators in the organization point to service excellence as a top priority. They ask department directors to support this priority and engage their staffs in pursuing it with energy and dedication.

With marching orders clear, managers proceed to communicate this priority to their staffs. But we have observed that very often, the tone, in contrast to the verbal message, thinly veils resistance to yet another institutional priority. Note how four managers communicate to their staff their commitment to service excellence:

> *Manager 1:* Staff, I want you to know that your administration has told us we're going to be pursuing service excellence here. They said that this is the wave of the future for hospitals and that we are supposed to get involved. They feel strongly that service excellence is the way to gain a competitive advantage in today's marketplace. They asked me to tell you about this.

> *Manager 2:* Staff, I'm so delighted to tell you that this hospital is going to focus on service excel-

lence as an important organizationwide priority.
I'm very happy about this because so many
people here need to improve their behavior
toward customers. Fortunately, the ambitious
organizationwide strategy won't be too demanding of us, because we already act the way others
should. I'm hoping that, at last, this service strategy will pull the rest of this hospital's staff to
where we've always been.

Manager 3: Thanks for taking this time out of
your extremely busy schedules. This won't take
long and then you can get back to the job. This
organization will be working to improve service
on everybody's parts. There will be a whole series
of events and new policies instituted to improve
service. I'm sorry that this will mean yet another
pressure on you who are already working so hard
with very lean staffing. I want to assure you that
I'll do all I can to make sure this service excellence strategy doesn't interfere with your job too
much and that we limit the time involved.

Manager 4: I want you to know that this organization is going to institute a service excellence
strategy. It's a good thing! Let's face it, behavior
is pretty bad. And, if we don't get our act together
in this place, we're going to be out of jobs. This
emphasis on service had better whip us into
shape!

All four managers avoided ownership of the forthcoming strategy. The first manager conveyed her belief that this
strategy was imposed by the administration. She was going
to cooperate because she was told to. This attitude reinforces
"we-they" feelings between the staff and the higher-ups who
are imposing this strategy.

The second manager agrees that service excellence is

important to the hospital, but then proceeds to exempt her staff from having to pay attention to it.

The third manager, fearful of asking anything more of his staff, apologizes for the imposition—for taking them "away from the job." He conveys his belief that this so-called organizationwide priority is not part of the job, but an additional burden. He even promises to protect his staff from it.

The fourth manager puts the blame on the external environment and uses punitive language to frighten staff into cooperation.

All four managers have failed to communicate their ownership of and commitment to the service excellence strategy. Envision the impact of their messages on staff motivation. All four managers undermine the service excellence strategy and generate staff resentment, not commitment. In the light of their managers' attitudes, staff are not likely to take the forthcoming strategy seriously or participate actively.

Ironically, all four managers would say that they had communicated to their staffs the importance of the forthcoming strategy. They did relay the news, but they certainly did not inspire staff to participate. In fact, all four managers provided staff with excuses for rejecting the change.

The preceding situations occurred; they are not exaggerated examples. Many managers have, albeit unintentionally, diminished the potential of change strategies by communicating their own resistance in subtle ways and increasing "we-they" sentiment.

What is needed instead? You must grapple with the new priority internally and find some way to commit to it, as did one manager:

> I want to let you know that our organization will be launching what I believe will be an exciting and important new priority. We're calling it a service excellence strategy. It's a strategy I think we've needed for a long time. We're going to launch an all-out focus on service for many reasons—the competitive environment and the need

to outshine our competitors by achieving unbeatable levels of satisfaction among our patients, physicians, and visitors. Also, since our patients are vulnerable, they deserve the quality of service and compassion that makes them feel special, secure, and in good hands.

I am also going to make sure that our focus on service extends to ourselves and our co-workers. In these stressful times, when we are all stretched to the limit, we need to pay special attention to the quality of interaction and support we extend to one another. In my view, that has to be an essential aspect of our service excellence strategy.

As I learn more about our strategy, I will keep you posted and I will look for ways every one of us can become actively involved. I am really excited about this and I hope you will be too.

Strategy 3: Help your staff walk in others' shoes. A significant way to build organizational perspective is to help employees view problems and events from different viewpoints, so that they can understand what other people in the organization think and feel.

It is easy to develop tunnel vision as we go about our daily routines. The more difficult our jobs, the harder it becomes to remain aware of and respect others' needs. This attitude may be easy to understand perhaps, but not easy to condone.

Tunnel vision fuels "we-they" thinking and makes effective teamwork unlikely. To strengthen cohesiveness and interdependence, people must be able to balance their own needs with the needs of others, and this requires the widened perspective acquired by walking in others' shoes.

You can help employees broaden their perspective by pushing them to understand and respect viewpoints of employees within and outside your department.

Many techniques exist to help employees widen their

perspective, for example, interdepartmental visitations, role swapping, and cross-training. You can also devote meeting time to helping staff experience new viewpoints. We illustrate here two such techniques that are extremely powerful: "the glass house" and "ideal versus real." These techniques require the services of a skilled group facilitator. If you lack such skills, ask for help from others in your organization with the necessary skills.

The Glass House. One way to help employees understand different points of view is to create a situation in which different groups can observe each other—"a glass house." Department meetings, workshops, retreats, any forum in which two groups (for example, administrators and department heads, nurses and pharmacists, lab personnel and unit secretaries, physicians and nurses) can be brought together can serve as a glass house.

1. Ask a few members from group A to form a small circle in the middle of the room. Ask the others from group A and all of group B to form a large circle surrounding the inner circle.
2. While members of the outer circle observe and listen silently, help members of the inner circle formulate answers to specific questions, for example, What is life like as a [your job] in this hospital? What makes it difficult to do your job? What do you wish others would understand about your job? What do you like most about being a [your job] in this hospital? What do you feel [a specific customer group] need most from you? Design the questions to raise awareness and heighten understanding. Or have one group generate questions for the other group ahead of time, to build greater personal investment.
3. Repeat this process several times, so that all convened have the chance to be part of the inner circle. You might also place an empty chair in the inner circle, so that a member from the outer circle with a burning question can join the circle, ask the question, and return immediately to the outer circle.

4. End by asking people to share what they learned about other people and other departments.

Ideal Versus Real. With the ideal-versus-real activity, you can also help employees learn more about each other and build mutual respect. Each group shares its vision of what the other group should be, and both groups work from there to negotiate realistic expectations. The following plan was implemented by technologists and radiologists in one hospital:

1. Separate groups with respect to position, so that technologists are seated together and physicians are seated together. Give each group a large piece of paper and a marker. Ask each group to brainstorm the characteristics of the *ideal* member of the other group. Technologists brainstorm a profile of the ideal radiologist, and radiologists brainstorm a profile of the ideal technologist.
2. After ten minutes, reconvene both groups to share their lists. The facilitator should make these points:
    A. Each group has expectations of the other. These expectations are based on many things. Yet, it is impossible for one group to meet all of the other group's expectations. Unfortunately, when expectations are not met, relationships are in jeopardy.
    B. This is an opportunity to clear the air and allow groups to share, even if they view this only as wishful thinking. Afterward, we will talk about what really is possible.
3. Now for reality. Explain that holding on to these ideal images can be damaging. Separate the groups again and ask them to set their standards of perfection aside and discuss what they most need and want from each other, as in these examples.
    A. Technologists may have envisioned the "perfect" radiologist as available to read films whenever the techs need them read. In reality, techs do need films read in a timely manner; when no one is available

to read them, patients are kept waiting. The two groups need to discuss and arrive at realistic, mutually workable expectations regarding timely reading of films.

B. Radiologists may have envisioned the "perfect" technologist as never taking a "bad" picture and, therefore, never wasting the radiologist's time. In reality, a few bad films are inevitable, but carelessness is frustrating, because everyone's time is consumed.

Give the separate groups enough time to discuss what they really need from one another. Then ask them to share what they believe to be realistic expectations with the other group.

4. Where do we go from here? Reunite the two groups and ask them to tag problems that merit further work. Subdivide into committees (representing both technologists and radiologists) to tackle some of these problems before a follow-up meeting.

5. End with a motivational pitch. Thank people for involving themselves in this difficult discussion and reinforce the need to continue building mutual respect.

Some people claim that organizational perspective is a thing of the past. It is true that in the past, people felt more secure about their jobs and the organization's commitment to them, and so it was easier to be loyal. Whether the manager's job is secure or not, thinking on behalf of the organization is required of managers at all levels. If you do not take the broader view about what is good for the organization, you are neglecting your responsibility and contributing to the divisiveness that tears organizations apart.

Now is the time to take the lead in healing the rifts that erode your organization's strength.

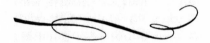

From Cynicism to Optimism

1. Do you think your colleagues find you obstructive in meetings? YES NO
2. Do you voice doubts about senior management in conversations with your employees? YES NO
3. Do you gripe about work at least weekly with colleagues? YES NO
4. Do you have a hard time forgiving others? YES NO
5. Do you see change as a threat more than an adventure? YES NO
6. Are you more likely to complain than to take action to make things better? YES NO
7. Do you think most managers in your organization think you are a positive force? YES NO
8. Would your colleagues consider you a cheerleader for the organization? YES NO
9. Do you think your employees regard you as openly appreciative of their efforts? YES NO
10. Do you avoid peers who complain often and unproductively? YES NO
11. Do you keep your employees motivated? YES NO

12. Do you help others see the good in the
    organization?   YES   NO

   If you answered "no" to the first six questions and "yes" to the last six questions you have an optimistic mind-set with respect to your work and the organization. "Yes" answers to the first six questions and "no" answers to the last six questions reflect a cynicism toward your work and the organization.

   Optimists tend to focus on the up side. They realize there are obstacles but believe they can overcome them. Instead of being pessimistic, they purport that a great deal is possible until proven otherwise. Optimists do not gravitate toward peers who gripe and complain. They avoid them, because they feel depleted when they associate with cynics. They also help others see the good around them—the strengths of the organization, the adventure in change, and the opportunity to play an important role in the organization.

   On the other hand, cynics tend to see the down side. They act as if very little is possible until proven otherwise and are quicker to complain and gripe than to take constructive action. They also are alert to obstacles. Unlike optimists, however, they cite obstacles as reasons for inaction and hang onto past resentments and disappointments. Cynics seek out others who openly make negative comments, resulting in the erosion of employee confidence in the organization.

Optimism: A Choice, Not a Fact

True or false? (1) Patients receive better health care now than they did five years ago. (2) Our health care system is better today than five years ago. There are no right answers. Your answers depend on your point of view.

   Consider the first statement: Patients receive better health care now than they did five years ago. Many people think that patients *have* received better health care recently because of the shift to more outpatient surgery and the resulting reduction in inpatient complications. Others think we have become more entrenched in a two-tiered health care system that gives rich people outstanding care, but provides poor people with no care at all. Still others feel that because of resource constraints, care is generally worse for everybody. Is there not a grain of truth in each of these positions?

Now, consider the second statement: Our health care system is better today than five years ago. Many consumers agree. They believe that the health care system has vastly improved because there are so many more alternatives. Also, health care organizations now focus on improving service quality to attract and retain patients. Consumers take better service quality as evidence that the system has improved, because they tend to judge quality on the basis of service criteria. But many hospital employees do not agree. They suffer the daily stress of staffing shortages, resource constraints, and insecurity. Many wonder how anyone of sound mind could think the health care system is better today than in the earlier days of stability and adequate staffing. Your position depends on your point of view.

The point is that you can *choose* the lens through which you view the complexity of our health care industry and the many facets of your own organization or department. The particular lens you choose has a powerful impact on your organization, your staff, your customers, and even your own job satisfaction and effectiveness. If you choose to see your world through a positive lens, you will see a positive work environment in which change is aimed at improvement. On the other hand, if you choose to see your world through a negative lens, you see problems, disappointments, frustrations, and obstacles.

Undoubtedly, you have recognized the power and the consequences of the lenses through which you and your staff view the organization. You probably know two nurses in similar situations whose worlds dramatically differ because of their perspectives. They have the same hours, the same boss, the same educational level, the same pay, and the same coworkers. One nurse sees the glass as half-empty; the other sees the glass as half-full. The cynic enervates co-workers, whereas the optimist spreads his or her attitude to co-workers.

The same is true for managers. Today, your organization needs optimists. Cynics deplete employees of energy, accomplish very little, erode pride and confidence in the organization, and block the forward movement necessary to compete effectively.

Today you cannot afford to focus on what you are losing: the constraints, the frustrations—the good old days. You need to focus on the windows of opportunity, to see barriers as challenges that dare you to stretch. You have the power to slough off cynicism on the part of others, when it drags you down. You do not have to conform to the prevailing negativity. You need to embrace optimism, so that you energize yourself and your staff to advance your organization's goals.

Consider the different approaches that stem from a cynical versus an optimistic stance in the following situations.

Case 1: Assume that your organization has to reduce staff. How would you discuss the cutbacks with the staff who remain? The cynic wallows in negativity and perhaps gripes about the organization, raising questions about the soundness of the administrators' judgment and competence. As a consequence, staff show decreased commitment, are insecure, lose their confidence, and revise their resumes in preparation for job hunting.

After explaining the painful facts, the optimist is more likely to stress that downsizing will result in a clearer focus on a smaller number of strong aspects of the organization and will afford the remaining staff greater visibility and more influence. This manager expresses confidence that the organization can meet the challenges ahead by being slim and trim.

Case 2: Because of a gigantic reduction in reimbursement to your hospital, the administration has just announced a series of deep budget cuts that affect your department. What do you say to your peers over coffee? The cynic lets his or her negativity show: "Can you believe we didn't get any input into that

decision! We're just lackeys around here who keep things
going and do all the work." The optimist is more likely to
feel sympathy for the administrators and seek the reasons for
the cuts so she or he can explain the situation to staff in
a way that maintains their maximum confidence in the
organization.

*Case 3: Physicians who deal with your department often
complain that it takes too long to get the information they need
from your department. You devise a way to reduce turnaround
time greatly, but your solution is expensive.* Some cynics pre-
judge that in the presence of resource constraints, funds for
reducing turnaround time will not be allocated, so they do
not even try to implement their plan. When confronted by
physicians, they explain that the situation is hopeless. Other
cynics may try halfheartedly to secure the funds, bringing the
problem to their boss's attention but not making a case for
the solution (that is, the positive consequences for the organization). The boss most likely will demand the details before
considering the allocation of funds. Cynics consider this response negative and discouraging, tantamount to rejection of
their proposal, and give up. Optimists, on the other hand,
go to the trouble of building a careful case to obtain the
resources they need to alleviate the problem with turnaround
time. They think, "Maybe this will work if I do my homework." They give it a try.

Optimism Versus Cynicism: The Consequences

At the very thought of "choosing" optimism, many managers
well up with resistance:

- It's easy for you to say. *Your* experience *is*
  positive.
- If you knew my situation, you would know
  how crazy optimism is.
- My friends would take me for a fool.
- I'm not going to be a naive pollyanna.

These reflections of resistance are understandable because numerous benefits are associated with cynicism. Cynics can blame other people and circumstances for their failure or inaction. As we all know, griping can be quite therapeutic. Cynics vent frustration and relieve personal stress by griping. Also, gripe sessions have immense social value. People are united against their common enemy. They feel powerful when they join together in their feeling of oppression.

Cynics also avoid "paying the price" that optimists pay. They do not run the risk of being called naive. They are so keenly attuned to worst-case scenarios they are unlikely to be disappointed. And, they cannot be accused of minimizing others' genuinely felt doubts, fears, frustrations, and concerns.

But cynics miss out on the benefits of optimism. Optimists report feeling upbeat and energetic, and even experience fewer diseases. They are more hopeful because they focus on the possibilities. They see improvements and solutions because they are open to them and persist until they find them. They are respected and appreciated by their bosses and suffer less turnover among their staffs because of their positive effects on morale. And, optimists are markedly more marketable in this day and age when organizations seek inspirational, forward-looking leaders to fill management positions.

In addition, optimists avoid "paying the price" that cynics pay. They are not called "nay sayers," "drags," and "bad mouthers." They do not spark depression among their colleagues. And they are not likely to ignore the good things happening around them, so they can feel successful and appreciative.

Strategies Aimed Toward a New Optimism

Optimism is a must today. Your point of view is highly contagious, especially to the people you manage. If you are a cynic, your staff will feel encouragement to voice their own doubts and gripes. If you are an optimist, your staff will be energized by your presence. If you truly believe that your situation is in every way too limiting or discouraging to warrant a realistic optimism, you will, because of your management position, legitimize that belief among staff. You will burn out—a victim of battle fatigue. Cynicism robs precious energy from you and those around you.

Your organization faces too many challenges to tolerate such behavior. Realistic optimism, not blind optimism, is a necessity. If you are a cynic, explore the ways in which you can move toward a more positive stance. If you cannot focus on the energizing aspects of your work or the organization, perhaps you should seriously consider leaving the organization before you are forced to.

Four strategies can help you alter your mindset and translate it into reality: (1) Dare to be positive in the face of negativity; confront others' cynicism. (2) Inject optimism at staff meetings. (3) Show positively your regard for individuals. (4) Establish a "free zone."

Strategy 1: Dare to be positive in the face of negativity; confront others' cynicism. Hospital XYZ, a teaching hospital, was concerned because of a decrease in the number of interns who chose this hospital for their residency. To diagnose the underlying problems that repelled prospective residents, the hospital conducted interviews with residents who chose a competitor hospital after considering Hospital XYZ. When asked why they had not chosen Hospital XYZ, several residents commented that during their visit to the hospital, the people they talked to (other residents, physicians, and staff) seemed negative about the organization. Puzzled by this, the researcher stopped current residents in the halls and elevators to ask why they had spoken so negatively about the hospital: "That's the way everybody talks here, even though we *like* this place." In other words, cynicism had become part of the culture—a habit, even though most employees thought the hospital was "a great place." Yet cynicism was having a detrimental effect on the organization, on morale, and on people's pride.

The only antidote was for individuals to question cynicism as an accepted mode of behavior in the organization's culture, to confront the negative comments and generalizations daily. If your organization has kneejerk cynics who are perceived as opinion leaders, you can be sure that there are closet optimists among you who feel alone and even a bit crazy. Help them out of the closet.

Confront cynicism and dare people to see the up side. Confronting cynicism requires assertive language and guts:

- I don't see things as bleak at all. Here's what I think.
- I think you're focusing on the dark side, when in fact, there are many good aspects to this situation. For instance . . .
- When you make cynical cracks about every new thing I try, I feel annoyed.
- There are certainly two ways to look at this situation. I'm going to focus on the positive aspects, because it gives me more energy. Frankly, I wish you would too.
- [To your staff] While the news is discouraging, we don't have to be passive in the face of it. I'm sure we have ways we can minimize the effects, if we consider the alternatives. Let's focus on what we can do, not what we can't do.

If your staff are cynics, act to build group commitment to a "new optimism." Assert your belief that cynicism is rampant and is having negative consequences for people and the organization. Ask your staff to signal one another when cynicism rears its debilitating head. Help them become more aware of cynicism in their everyday language, by working with them to stamp out the "killer phrases and gestures."

You can push for optimism by employing the following activity at a staff meeting: Describe the evidence of cynicism and your perception of its destructive effects. Explain why you think optimism (wearing a positive lens) is a *choice* every individual has. Ask staff for their active involvement in building a "new optimism." Get them first to identify "killer phrases and gestures" and then to agree to help each other replace these with language and gestures that reflect the new optimism. Engage staff in brainstorming killer phrases and gestures. Then ask them to brainstorm constructive alternatives. Decide on a signal they can use to alert one another when they engage in a negative behavior (for example, raising a red flag or saying "bong"). Express appreciation for the support you anticipate.

Confronting cynicism among co-workers at any level takes guts; however, the alternative is to push endlessly against resistance and cynicism whenever you want to act or get others to act.

Strategy 2: Inject optimism at staff meetings. Encourage a spirit of optimism by institutionalizing attention to the positives in your staff meetings. The following quick aids for staff meetings reinforce optimism as a desired norm in your work environment.

Open staff meetings by asking all group members to answer one or more of the following questions: What is one good thing that happened to me this week? When I think about our division, what do I feel *good* about? What works well in our department?

Pose the question, What's good about now? People either can write nonstop for two minutes individually or brainstorm as a group and summarize their results. Rigidly enforce one ground rule: nothing negative.

Create ritual openings and closings to meetings (or work weeks) that nudge staff to focus on the positives around them. For example, What good things have occurred since we last met (accomplishments, events, news, activities, and the like)? and Let us end by reviewing what we have accomplished and what people have found gratifying about this week/meeting. Five minutes of optimism at the beginning and end of a meeting or a week reinforce a positive perspective.

Strategy 3: Show positively your regard for individuals. When the pressure is on, it is easy to focus on staff weaknesses because these do affect productivity and the effectiveness of the entire operation. Consequently, managers lose sight of or take for granted positive performance.

If you are prone to this attitude, consider techniques for ensuring that staff receive the positive recognition that human beings need to remain motivated. Appreciation telegrams (for use with individuals) and strength bombardment (for use with peers) are two such effective approaches.

Appreciation telegrams are vehicles by which patients, physicians, and staff show their appreciation for one another in writing. Devise a format similar to that shown in Exhibit 8 that staff can use to recognize teamwork and special feats.

Exhibit 8. Appreciation Telegram.

To: Ann Jones

From: Hanna Brown, Department Director

Heard you worked wonders during Melissa Curran's traumatic delivery of her son. The Currans were so grateful for your attentiveness, support, and resourcefulness. They felt that they were in very good hands. I really appreciate all you do to make our patients satisfied customers. Thank you!

Strength bombardment promotes recognition and support among peers. Everyone in the group focuses on one person and bombards that person with positive feedback. Here is how it works:

- Write each employee's name on an index card. Scramble the cards in a box or hat. Ask employees (maximum of twenty) to sit in a circle. Leave one empty chair, the "spotlight chair," in the middle of the circle.
- Explain to your group how strength bombardment works. You will select one card at a time. The person whose name is picked sits in the spotlight chair. For one full minute, the rest of the group bombards this staff member with positive feedback: strengths, contributions to the department, admirable personality traits, ability to work with others, and so on.

- Continue to spotlight individuals until each person has had a turn. Do not include a card with your name. Wait for someone to recognize that you have not had a turn and then take the spotlight. If this does not happen, do not be disappointed. It is not wise to put employees on the spot with their boss.
- Solicit reactions to the exercise by inviting quick responses to these questions: How did it feel to give recognition? How did it feel to receive recognition?

Strategy 4: Establish a "free zone." Your staff need a "free zone," a safe place in which you will listen to their concerns openly and nondefensively. The venting of negative feelings is therapeutic as long as you and your staff do not dwell on the negative but act to formulate solutions. Therefore, designate a time and place for constructive venting. In some hospitals, managers allow for venting at brown-bag lunches. Without such an arrangement, cynicism will build and cause great damage.

Two free zones are the "sound off" meeting and the old-fashioned complaint box.

In a sound-off meeting, the manager invites employees to voice their opinion of the strengths of the department, as well as their problems and frustrations. The manager sets three ground rules: (1) There will be no name calling. (2) Participation must be widespread. (3) People must listen to and accept others' feelings, even if they have a different perception. First, the staff brainstorms the "positives," for example, projects that are going well, procedures that work, positive feelings about work. These are listed on a flipchart or chalkboard. Then the staff brainstorms the "negatives," for example, procedures that do not work, frustrations, factors that interfere with job satisfaction.

No one person should dominate the meeting. You, as the manager, should be a role model of effective, nondefensive listening. At the end, work with the group to divide the problems mentioned into three lists, depending on the type of follow-up needed: (1) Nothing can be done. (2) Nothing can be done at this time, but we will review it at a specified date in the future. (3) This problem needs attention and problem solving and here is who will work on it. Thank people for their openness and announce what you as manager will do in the way of follow-up.

Also install in an accessible place a box for complaints. Attach a pen and tablet, making it easy for people to write while on the run. Promise a *timely* response.

True, times are tough. But to make the best of them, focus on what is happening and what is possible—the accomplishments, the service provided, the healed patients, the productive staff, the support available, the problems solved, the revenue earned, the exciting plans, experimentation, innovation, and more. Your organization's future rests on it.

Until recently, hospitals were orderly organizations with clear procedures, sufficient funds, functional rules, and a relatively unruffled pecking order. Patients advanced along settled paths. This order has been replaced by not only noise, confusion, scrambling in every direction, and perhaps a lot of wasted energy but also flexibility, opportunity, and, if you choose to see it that way, adventure.

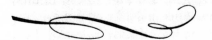

Gaining Organizational Support for Making Role Changes

In Chapters Two to Eleven, we examined ten role shifts that can make you indispensable to your organization. You can demonstrate both the willingness and the ability to fulfill these new role demands; however, as you do not operate in a vacuum, you might not be able to do it alone.

Some executive teams and some health care cultures are ready for managers to function in new ways and even encourage them, through word and deed, to make the necessary transitions. In other organizations, however, managers who want to contribute actively and set the pace for progress encounter barrier after barrier. When these managers do what senior management claims to want, the consequences are negative.

Of course, your ability to be successful in your role depends partly on people, policies, practices, incentives, and environmental circumstances. To expedite your transition, you can benefit greatly from, first, the absence of impediments, and second, outright support from your boss, your organization, and your peers.

In this chapter, we examine forces that block managers

180

in their efforts to embrace new role demands and outline the types of support you need to increase your effectiveness. For each of the ten role shifts, we identify at least one specific form of support your own boss can supply and suggest how you can secure this support if it is not forthcoming. You may well have to become proactive in educating senior management to provide you with the support you need to fulfill their expectations and achieve the results they desire. They, too, have operated in a different culture and, more often than not, need help reshaping their own role in relation to you.

We also explore the forms of support the organization can and should provide (for example, structures and growth opportunities) to nurture strength and resilience within your organization's entire management team.

Support, Shift by Shift

Adopt a Customer Orientation. Customer-oriented managers agree on what they need most from their bosses to translate their customer orientation into reality. When they make a compelling case for resources, a case that shows greater benefits than costs to the organization, they need to know that they will get those resources. Managers tell us that they follow their organization's process for proposing improvements in customer service and that even when the need is obvious and meticulously justified, it is ignored without reason. It is true that managers must learn to be creative in extending the resources available; doing more with less is a business necessity. If customer satisfaction is truly a priority, however, resources must be released for necessities like adequate staffing and flexible scheduling. And, executives need to give managers answers in a timely fashion when these managers have done all they can at their level. Why should managers elicit and examine customer feedback, strategically build a departmental service culture, be creative about satisfaction enhancement strategies, and monitor and coach employees to satisfy customers, if resources are unavailable.

If you are failing to get the support you need to become

more customer oriented, then confront your boss. If you have documented the need and the solution, and the benefits outweigh the costs, then ask your boss when he or she will give you answer. Your boss may still say, "That's just how it is," admitting his or her own powerlessness. At least you will know you did your part.

The powers-that-be need to provide responses and sometimes resources when you make a convincing case. Otherwise, your imagination and energy will dim.

Raise and Maintain Higher Standards. To institute and enforce higher standards related to employee performance, you need support from your personnel department and your boss when you confront employees who do not meet these higher standards. Without this backup, why should you confront employees? We have heard from many managers who have followed the proper procedure (clarify expectations, document behavior) only to hear "Try again. Try to work with this employee. We don't want to get rid of this person, because they know the president of our board [or they've been here a long time, or they have a sick mother]!" or the manager is seen as the problem, because the personnel file does not indicate performance problems in the past. So either you are pressured to try again or the employee is transferred to another department and you feel guilty.

To hold employees accountable to higher standards, you need assurance that senior management wants higher standards too and that if you do your homework, your personnel decisions will be supported.

If your administration does not support enforcement of higher standards and if your human resources department is known for "never firing anyone," outline the process you propose to use to hold a problem employee accountable, check over the process with your boss, articulate the possibility that you might need his or her support, and ask outright for their commitment to back you up in the event of a problem. Also ask your boss to serve as an intermediary between you and human resources if you anticipate a problem there.

With respect to safety, security, clinical care, equipment performance, and the like, your organization must provide you with the tools to meet higher standards. If these are not available, once again you must confront senior management with the reality that higher standards are unattainable unless the tools are available. Go a step further. Determine which tools you need and, instead of telling your superior that it is impossible to meet the high standard, say, "You and I both want to meet this higher standard. To do so, we need the following. I have looked into the options and here is what it will entail." Show your commitment to the standard and help senior management provide what is needed.

Empower Employees. Consider two pieces of middle management folklore:

It's not my place to run the train; the whistle I can't blow.

It's not my place to say how far the train's allowed to go.

It's not my place to shoot off steam or even clang the bell.

But let the damn thing jump the track and see who catches hell.

Around here, I have a very responsible position. Whenever anything goes wrong, I'm responsible.

You cannot empower employees if you do not have power yourself. Yet, many managers feel powerless. You must be able to make decisions concerning your department without obtaining permission from superiors at every step. Managers complain that their hands are tied, or that when they are free to act decisively, they are reprimanded if they make a mistake.

If this situation sounds familiar, talk it over with your boss. Just as you might have a problem giving up control, so might your boss. Describe the instances when you felt your initiative was thwarted. Find out what you can do to ease your boss's fears about loosening the reins, for example, keep him or her informed more thoroughly and routinely. If your boss refuses to give you a blanket approval, see if together you can work out categories of decisions you *can* make. Be specific. Provide sample situations in which you want to make decisions without permission.

As you can be sure your boss also suffers from overload, remind her or him that delegation of more responsibility to you would be efficient and would reduce his or her work load. Reassure your boss that you will study the implications of your decisions carefully. The point is if you want rope, ask for it. And if you do not get it, confront your boss and discuss how you both can move toward a stronger partnership of mutual trust within which you have latitude to act.

Treat Your Employees as Customers. Just as you need to nurture employees to increase their effectiveness, win their dedication and loyalty to you and the organization, and thus retain them, so must senior management pay similar attention to you. Yet managers report that the higher one rises, the rarer it is to receive a pat on the back. If your boss fails to acknowledge you, you can bet that he or she feels unappreciated. As one CEO said, "I don't get positive feedback from my cohorts or the board or doctors. The only way I know if I'm doing a good job in their eyes is if they let me keep my job."

That might be the harsh reality, but it does not motivate managers. If you feel unappreciated, figure out the accomplishment for which you want to be appreciated. Then, *ask* your boss for feedback. Do not wait for your boss to provide it. Also ask peers for feedback and become the role model of the nurturing manager.

Become Proactive. To take the initiative, you require information to ensure that your initiatives are appropriate. And you need support in the form of feedback from your boss. If every project you begin, if every idea you generate, if every proposal you write is shelved, your enthusiasm will surely waver.

You especially need someone to run interference for you, to clear the red tape, so that you can reach the right person, find the needed information, and move forward without impediments.

To get such support from your boss, make sure that every meeting with your boss ends with a concrete plan of action. Proactively outline the steps and facilitate the process, instead of leaving decisions hanging.

Experiment and Take Risks. Of all the role shifts, this is the one frequently discouraged, often in subtle but nonetheless powerful ways. So many health care organizations have been risk-averse that many senior managers are themselves steeped in risk aversion. Therefore, when you experiment and take risks, you might well get your hands slapped.

A thick skin helps, but so does some semblance of support from the organization. Higher-ups need to extend to you the freedom to take risks and experiment, make mistakes, and learn from these mistakes without repercussion. They must let you know that you are valued, respected, and capable and that your judgment is sound. No manager goes out on a limb unless he or she believes it is "reasonably" safe to do so. Also, your boss needs to point out your mistakes to you (if you are not aware of them) to improve your batting average but not kill your spirit. The boss must clarify what worked, what did not work, and what can be done differently the next time. Then, and here is the hard part for many, your boss needs to thank you for taking the risk on behalf of the organization and express the hope that you will continue to do so in the future.

If your boss has actively discouraged risk taking and experimentation, consider bottom-up coaching. Share with your boss how you have encouraged your people to take risks and the results. Describe the language you used to encourage them before and after successes and failures. Teach by example. Or, in the spirit of risk taking, come right out and ask your boss for support, articulating exactly what type of support you want. Share with your boss your feelings about punitive feedback for past risks and its dampening effect on your initiative.

These suggestions entail confrontation. And some senior managers do not welcome or even tolerate confrontation. Assert yourself tactfully, so, at the least, you will know you did all you could. If the support is then withheld or matters are made worse, the message to you is clear.

Emphasize Results. The greatest aid to a results-oriented manager is a boss who will help you fight the battles that you are not in a position to fight because of organizational politics and lines of authority.

You also need a boss who helps you remain focused on results—who outlines the results expected, who lets you know what you are being held accountable for. To help your boss, share your plans, hopes, and outcomes. Ask your boss to run interference for you when you are stumped.

Build Organizational Perspective. To develop a team that feels committed to the organization, you need *the cold, hard facts.* Information is power. You need to know the reasons for decisions and the implications for financial viability, quality, customer satisfaction, and the organization's future. Whether the information concerns implementation of a new procedure or explanation of a change in policy, you must understand the information you present to your people.

If you do not get the information you need, press for it. Waiting for senior management to recognize your need is not only inexcusably passive, but also ineffective. Take the risk and make your needs known. One manager made it very clear when asked to deliver news to her staff: "How would you like me to share this? What should I say are the reasons? What are the processes and by when will this be taking effect? I expect my staff to be upset about this because . . . I will try to avert their concern by saying . . . Is there any other way you want me to represent you and your decision in a positive light and in a way that builds employee confidence?"

Difficult? Absolutely, but this is one area where you cannot afford to be unclear. You must help your boss produce and share the information you need to build loyalty and organizational perspective among your staff.

Promote Teamwork. Two obstacles interfere with managers who want to cross departmental lines and work with other managers.

First, it is hard to promote teamwork among your staff when you do not feel that you are part of a team. How can you make your staff understand others' perspectives when the norm in the organization is "to mind your own business." Your boss needs to publicly support his or her own team and actively promote the rest of the organization. You cannot get caught in the middle of a turf war among top executives. Managers need a cohesive, open, administrative team, a team that spurs them to new heights of teamwork and interdepartmental initiatives.

If teamwork is not a norm in your organization, let your boss know how you and other managers think team spirit and interdepartmental problem solving can be developed. Propose solutions and find support among your peers in presenting those solutions to senior management.

The second, and we believe the most serious, impediment to teamwork among managers is the threat perceived by senior managers. After an exciting management team "renewal retreat," one group of department heads decided to hold an optional brown-bag lunch every week at which they could share accomplishments, problems, and needs. They were very enthusiastic about these self-motivated, self-run meetings. But then the CEO felt threatened or, as most managers recount, paranoid. He issued an edict that these meetings could not take place unless senior management was present. The impact? The well-intentioned managers were furious, claiming, rightfully so, that distrust and suspicion from the top breeds distrust and suspicion across department lines.

If senior management asks staff to act as a team but then views them as subversive when they do, schedule a meeting with the CEO in which supportive department heads (there is safety in numbers) tactfully share their perceptions of team-building initiatives and the negative impact of suspicion and interference by senior management.

Finally, if you believe something dramatic is needed to turn the tide, recommend to your administrators that an off-site team-building retreat be held with all managers in attendance. Suggest that an outside facilitator be hired who can interview people without bias and tailor an intervention customized to the organization. Sell it to senior management by spelling out the benefits of reduced organizational stress, more cooperation between departments, and greater communication throughout the organization.

Be an Optimist. It certainly helps to have a boss who does not harp on problems and obstacles, but instead attends to accomplishments and possibilities. A positive executive spreads her or his enthusiasm and consequently energizes and inspires staff. By setting the stage, senior management allows you to focus on the good and the possible without appearing foolish in front of your people.

How can you get executives to "stop and smell the roses"? Ask for time out at a management meeting and spend several minutes looking at the positives. Or, suggest to top management that a key executive share with the management team a positive vision of the organization and the challenges ahead.

Finally, set in motion from the ground up your own policy of emphasizing the positive and confronting negativity. One manager expressed the following:

> Our management team, top and middle, was a mess. All anyone did was complain and focus on the negative. If you spoke up or said anything positive, you were an outcast. Finally, several of us got together and examined the effect this nega-

tivity was having on us and others. We started an optimism campaign calling ourselves the new optimists.

We approached top management with the idea of circulating a memo starting a war on negativity. They endorsed our proposal and agreed to support our efforts, but the proposal, campaign, and ideas were ours. We managers had had enough.

As a result, it became uncool and uncouth to be negative or unsupportive. In fact, managers were encouraged to signal (say "Bong" to) anyone who strayed from the new optimism.

A Supportive Organization

There are additional forms of support your organization can and should provide to spark your success and continued growth as a willing and able manager.

What can executives do to exercise their important responsibility of developing and sustaining a strong management team? Nothing fancy, really. They can serve as role model, make clear their expectations of managers, communicate openly, provide training and development opportunities, offer constructive feedback and coaching, hold managers accountable for embracing the new behavior, and reshape incentives and recognition practices to encourage willing and able managers to achieve new heights of energy and accomplishment.

Serve as a Role Model. Executives who want their managers to behave differently must model the desired behavior. Imagine the dissonance created when senior management asks middle managers to take risks and initiative, to communicate more openly, and to become proactive, while they remain risk-averse, passive in the face of change, and noncommunicative. They fail to be mentors to managers at lower levels. Every senior manager needs to be a role model.

Clarify Expectations of Managers. If your executive team wants you to make the ten role shifts examined in this book, they should be explicit. They should communicate to you their expectations and build these into your job descriptions. And they should work with you to achieve them. We have found that most managers move to fulfill expectations once they are made clear.

Communicate Openly. Managers need some direction, a sense of the big picture, and specific structures that ensure the continuous flow of information up, down, and across levels and positions. Although open, regular communication is everyone's responsibility, it is up to senior management to establish the channels of communication—department management meetings, cluster groups, typed minutes of executive and management meetings, internal newsletters, breakfasts with the boss, rap sessions, focus groups, and others.

Provide Training and Development Opportunities. New roles demand new skills. Your organization should provide training and development that will help you flex your management muscles and expand your style and skills. Whether through tuition reimbursement or in-house training programs, a laboratory in which you can learn and try new skills and approaches is a must. Executives who believe they cannot afford such programs pay dearly in the long run.

Offer Constructive Feedback and Coaching. It is not enough to be judged annually in a performance appraisal. You must be told when you have gone too far or not far enough and when you have handled specific people and situations inappropriately. New roles demand new behavior, and you deserve feedback and individual tutelage before the ax falls.

Hold Managers Accountable for Embracing the New Behavior. If senior management does not hold you accountable to new role demands, the word "demands" becomes moot. Change is tough and most people resist it. After being coached and counseled, managers who fail to meet the demands of their new role must change. If they do not change and are allowed to stay, senior management is merely providing a sanctuary for unwilling and unable managers who drag down the organization and dampen morale.

Reshape Incentives and Recognition Practices. The carrot, not just the stick, must be there when managers rise to new heights. Willing and able managers deserve rewards, bonuses, acknowledgment, new challenges, promotions, and opportunities.

You do need support to sustain effective changes in your role, but you should not wait for it. Start now. Act to make the changes, and if the rhetoric is there without the support, become an activist. Seek support, freedom to act, responsibility, and information. Through your own behavior, send ripples through your organization. If you see no hope for support in your present situation even after your efforts to obtain it, your options are clear: revert to your old ways, build peer support and try to change your organization from the middle, remain the lone maverick with all its accompanying tension, or leave the organization for another that welcomes your initiative and leadership.

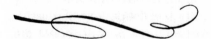

13

Achieving Personal and Organizational Success

As you read this book, you probably measured yourself against the role shifts presented. We hope you found validation for the roles you already play. Perhaps you identified pathways that will lead you to increase your management effectiveness. We also hope we have convinced you that the question is not whether to change, but how to change. Many options are available; doing nothing is hardly one of them.

We asked four managers with different styles who feel they have successfully made these role shifts to reflect on their experience:

The Dragged

> I worked there for thirty-two years. I was there through one administration after another. I heard everybody say how they were going to change things and how they wanted new energy from us managers. I nodded politely, knowing full well that we would run like crazy—in place. I learned to wait it out and managed the way I always did.

Then, we got a new administrator and she went all out to build a top management team. She told us in no uncertain terms that we had to start running the place, that, with new ventures, board and physician relations, managed care plans, and the like, she just would not be able to stay on top of operations. She pushed us to get off the dime. I watched, thinking she too would come and go. But she did not and some of my colleagues—and even diehards like me—started to get more involved. I started to feel like an outsider and wonder if maybe I was digging my own grave. I guess that is when I started to listen and to change. I knew that it was change or else. And I have changed, even though I had to be dragged kicking and screaming.

The Surfer

I'm a "follower" type of person. I go with the tide. When other department heads started to take more initiative and get some good results and some recognition from higher-ups, that is when I found myself changing. It was like getting swept up in a current.

The Gradualist

I liked the idea of making these changes. To tell you the truth, the new way is the way I thought it would be when I first became a manager. But of course it was not and I learned to manage for the status quo. Now that the environment is changing, I need to relearn. I am one of those people that goes slowly, that feels my way instead of barging right in. I will change in my own time.

The Existential Leaper

> It was sort of like standing on the edge of a freez-
> ing pool. You try to get your nerve to jump in.
> When you cannot, you dip your big toe and wait
> until it gets used to the water. You keep telling
> yourself that if your toe can get used to it, the
> rest of you can too. Then, you pull back and give
> yourself a pep talk like "Grow up; stop being a
> baby." This goes on until finally you just jump.
> And within a matter of moments, you find that
> you not only are used to it, but it is refreshing
> and invigorating. That describes my experience
> changing my approach to management.

There are no doubt other approaches to personal change as
well.

You can change if you choose to, in your own way.
Whether gradually or suddenly, you can embrace the role
changes key to your viability and success as a health care
manager.

To clarify the best next steps for you, create your own
agenda for change:

1. Assess your strengths and weaknesses in relation to the
    role shifts presented.
2. Set your personal priorities for change. You are un-
    doubtedly where you want to be in relation to some role
    shifts and not where you want to be in relation to
    others.
3. Consider your internal and external supports.
    A. What is there about *you* that will enable you to
        make your desired changes without undue pain or
        negative consequences? Your intelligence? Your com-
        mitment to health care? Your openness to feedback?
        Your sense of humor? List your internal strengths
        and be ready to call on them when you need per-
        spective or an anchor in rough seas.

B. Outside of yourself, who will support you during your change process? Who will provide honest feedback, encouragement, empathy, or even a respite from the stress involved? Your boss? Professional colleagues outside your organization? Peers within? Your staff? Senior management? A management support group you can create? A mentor? Friends and family? Written reinforcements in the form of favorite books and articles? Consider going public with the supportive people in your life. Tell them about the changes you are trying to make and educate them about what they can do to help.

4. Now, think through the obstacles to your changing, both internal and external.

A. Start by looking within yourself. Is the enemy within? Do your attitudes and habits work for or against you? Believe that these are malleable, and, perhaps by using the exercises described in this book, modify them to serve you better.

B. What about the external obstacles—an unsupportive boss, double messages from senior management, colleagues who treat you as a member of the lunatic fringe? Confront them. Tell them your goals and let them know how their words, actions, and inaction affect you adversely. This might be news to them, and helpful news at that.

5. Create your strategy. Determine sensible first steps in your effort to change. Decide which new behavior you want to try first and identify situations at work that provide you with the opportunity to try this behavior.

6. Go public with your plan. Involve others—your boss, your staff, your friends. Their support helps you and also puts some pressure on you to follow through.

7. Finally, figure out some way to monitor your progress. Ask others for feedback. Develop a checklist you can use to take stock of how you are doing, or compose a brief survey that your boss, staff, and peers can use to rate you on the roles you are trying to fulfill.

If you implement your personal agenda for change, you will most likely succeed in expanding your managerial behavior, because you do have the power to change. If, however, after making the changes you find yourself inhibited and discouraged by your boss or organization, you must face the fact that your organization is hostile to the very management behavior that is called for in the turbulent health care environment.

If mediocrity is not just tolerated but encouraged, if you do not have the freedom to make or learn from failures, if risk taking is squelched, if open criticism and confrontation are taboo, if your organization lacks a sense of direction, if teamwork is seen as subversive, then you face a much larger question. You have assessed your situation and concluded that sustained change is impossible, and if you still want to change and grow, you will need to look elsewhere to find an organization that supports and encourages your energy and initiative. You should seriously consider this possibility, because hospitals that foster stagnation will surely lose ground in today's competitive environment.

We persist in believing that you can change if you choose to and that your future as a health care manager depends on your ability to fulfill increasingly ambitious role demands. There are many payoffs: an end to questions about the worth and utility of your position; viability, credibility, and longevity in your management role; heightened respect for your innovations, solutions, and contributions to quality; results and accomplishments you can point to and take pride in; organizational progress as a result of your impact; and personal rejuvenation.

You should not have to worry about keeping your job. You should not be treated like deadwood because you manage for a nostalgic past. You should not plod along unchallenged and ineffectively because you shy away from opportunities to increase your contribution to your organization.

As a health care professional, you can and must do better than that. Expanding and stretching in the face of new role demands is a win-win situation. Health care organizations win because they compete more effectively in the capable hands of managers who exemplify and inspire peak performance. And you win because your new role is stimulating and gratifying. Stagnation is impossible.

In conclusion, some managers watch things happen. Others make things happen. And still others wonder what happened. Have the audacity to be a manager who makes things happen.

References

Bellman, G. M. "The Staff Manager as Leader." *Training,* 1988, 25 (2), 39–45.

Bradford, D. L., and Cohen, A. R. *Managing for Excellence.* New York: Wiley, 1984.

Deal, T. E., and Kennedy, A. A. *Corporate Cultures: The Rites and Rituals of Corporate Life.* Reading, Mass.: Addison-Wesley, 1982.

Einstein Consulting Group. *The Service Matrix.* Philadelphia: Einstein Consulting Group, 1986.

Einstein Consulting Group. *Service Quality Improvement Process.* Philadelphia: Einstein Consulting Group, 1989.

Herzberg, F. "One More Time: How Do You Motivate Employees?" *Harvard Business Review,* Sept.–Oct. 1987, pp. 109–120.

Lawler, E. E. "Transformation from Control to Involvement." In R. H. Kilmann and T. J. Covin (eds.), *Corporate Transformation: Revitalizing Organizations for a Competitive World.* San Francisco: Jossey-Bass, 1987.

Lawler, E. E., Renwick, P. A., and Bullock, R. J. "Employee Influence on Decisions: An Analysis." *Journal of Occupational Behavior,* 1981, 2, 115–123.

Le Boeuf, M. *The Greatest Management Principle in the World.* New York: Berkley Books, 1985.

Leebov, W. *Service Excellence: The Customer Relations Strategy for Health Care.* Chicago: American Hospital Publishing, 1988.

Maccoby, M. *Why Work?* New York: Simon & Schuster, 1988.

Peters, T. *Thriving on Chaos.* New York: Knopf, 1987.

Pinchot, G. *Intrapreneuring.* New York: Harper & Row, 1985.

Index

and experimentation, 109-110; for managers, 10-19; monitoring, 195; rapidity of, 106-107; support for, 194-195

Chrysler, failure and change at, 106

Coaching: bottom-up, 185-186; for empowerment, 73-76; for managers, 190

Cohen, A. R., 9

Communication: lines of, and empowerment, 72; of new expectations, 53-54; open, 190; for organizational view, 156-164

Competition, increasing, 3

Complaint box, and optimism, 179

Consultation, mutual, for teamwork, 142, 144-145

Co-Worker House Rules, 85-86

Creativity, exercising, 115-118

Culture: and customer orientation, 32-35; cynicism, 174-175; forces affecting, 33-35

Customer: as demanding, 2-3; employee as, 77-89; needs of, and results orientation, 128-130

Customer orientation: aspects of shift to, 20-39; attributes of, 23; background on, 21-23; benefits of, 26-27; cases showing, 23-25; and culture, 32-35; cyclical service management process for, 36-37; feedback for, 28-32; and management practices, 39; organizational support for, 181-182; self-assessments for, 20-21, 33-35; staff meetings for, 36, 38-39; and standards, 41; strains in, 25-26; strategies for, 27-39

Cutbacks. *See* Downsizing

Cyclical service management process, for customer orientation, 36-37

Cynicism: attributes of, 169; benefits of, 173; confronting, 174-176

D

Deal, T. E., 9

Decision Worksheet, 49-50

Delegation, and proactive behavior, 98

Delta Airlines, employee empowerment at, 72

Detroit, managers' responses in, 7

Divergent thinking, and experimentation, 115-116

Downsizing: customer orientation to, 23-24; memo confirming, 160; and optimism, 171

E

Efficiency, and experimentation, 109

Einstein Consulting Group, 29, 36

Employee Satisfaction Survey, 89

Employees: aspects of satisfaction for, 77-89; background on, 78-79; baggage of, 96-97; cases supporting, 80-81; empowering, 59-76; feedback to, and results orientation, 126, 130; group health responsibilities of, 88; hygiene and motivation factors for, 82; interrelationships of, 85-86; and language of appreciation, 83, 86, 88; and managerial types, 79-81; and managers, 150-151; monitoring satisfaction of, 88-89; needs of, 78-79, 82-83; organizational support for, 184; organizational view for, 164-167; self-assessment on, 77-78; shortage of, 5-6, 78, 92; standard raising involvement of, 57-58; strategies for loyalty of, 82-89; strengths of, and optimism, 176-178; and team building, 83-85; values changing among, 3-4. *See also* Staff meetings

Empowering staff: aspects of, 59-76; attributes of, 61; background on, 60-61; backup systems for, 70-73; barriers to, 63-64; benefits of, 64; cases practicing for, 68-69; cases showing, 62-63; coaching for, 73-76; input opportunities for, 65-68; judgment training for, 68-70; organizational support

ISBN 1-55542-248-9

90000